THE ART OF
HAIR WORK

Hair Braiding and Jewelry of Sentiment
with Catalog of Hair Jewelry
by
Mark Campbell
as supplemented with
Excerpts from Godey's Lady's Magazine

edited by
Jules & Kaethe Kliot

LACIS
PUBLICATIONS

3163 Adeline Street, Berkeley, CA 94703

© 1989, Jules Kliot
Second Printing, 1994

ISBN 0-916896-31-5

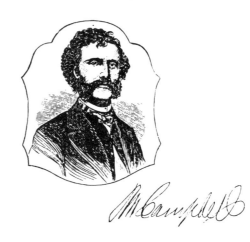

NEW EDITION.

SELF-INSTRUCTOR

IN THE

ART OF HAIR WORK

DRESSING HAIR,

Making Curls, Switches, Braids,

AND

HAIR JEWELRY OF EVERY DESCRIPTION.

Compiled from Original Designs and the Latest Parisian Patterns

BY

MARK CAMPBELL.

NEW YORK AND CHICAGO.

MDCCCLXXV.

Original Frontpiece, 1875

CONTENTS

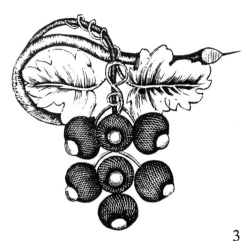

INTRODUCTION

The fascination of hair as a decorative and ornamental substance can be documented as early as the Egyptian era, where the immortality of human hair gave credence to finding the immortality of the body itself.

The Victorian era, with its roots in sentimentality, inspired new heights in the development of hair as an ornamental and coveted substance. As mementos of deceased as well as symbols of love and friendship, hair was placed in lockets, made into floral forms and braided for keepsakes of both the living and dead. Elaborate wreaths were formed from these forms and set in deep frames as remembrances.

The height of sophistication of hair work, however occurred mid 19th c. when elaborate hair jewelry or "jewelry of sentiment" as it was referred to, combined complex braids and gold findings to create decorative pins, rings, bracelets, necklaces, earrings and other items valued far more then if of pure gold work. It was a period of romanticizing, and the hair of a loved one was the perfect vehicle to express this bond of love.

While hair could be purchased, the import of such reaching hundreds of tons per year by mid 19th c., it was the personal association with the hair employed that had the most significance. Selected hair would be sent to the hair braiders and returned in the appropriately selected configuration.

While the specific techniques have been credited to European origins, they were to become a drawing-room occupation in Victorian America by the 1850's when the leading women's magazines, viz. *Lady Godey's* and *Petersons*, promoted the hair work crafts through many articles and patterns. The first book describing the techniques was not to come about till 1875 when Mark Campbell, revealed the secrets of over 100 designs in his book titled THE ART OF HAIR WORK.

Virtually identical in technique to the ancient Japanese braiding form known as *Kumi Himo*, which has been documented as early as the 9th c., no evidence has been found to connect 19th c. Victorian hair braiding with that of the Japanese which used silk as the working material. The Victorian technique seems to have developed independently of this Oriental influence, its origins in central Europe.

Most of the hair designs are unique, with methods unheard of in the Kumi Himo forms. The hair work patterns were of pure textural design, using openwork, shape and texture as the design elements. *Kumi Himo*, on the other hand relies primarily on texture and color, with the braids worked tight and dense. The hair working tools were of entirely different form and design, and in many ways far less elaborated then the Kumi Himo stands and looms.

The commercial making of hair jewelry survived well into the 20th c. with known locations in both in the US and Sweden as late as the 1960's when ads could still be found promoting hair jewelry as "a personal keepsake." To our knowledge there are no commercial makers of hair jewelry today, although with the resurgence of interest in kumi himo as well as interest and revival in Victorian Crafts, these elaborate braids and the working with hair would again seem to be timely.

The source for this edition of the *ART OF HAIR WORK* is the

**NEW EDITION
SELF-INSTRUCTOR IN THE ART OF HAIR WORK.
DRESSING HAIR, MAKING CURLS, SWITCHES, BRAIDS
AND HAIR JEWELRY
OF EVERY DESCRIPTION
COMPILED FROM ORIGINAL DESIGNS
AND THE LATEST PARISIAN PATTERNS
by Mark Campbell,**

published by the author in 1875. All references to hair braiding and jewelry have been retained, with the references to dressing hair omitted. This work is supplemented by material from the monthly **GODEY'S LADY'S BOOK AND MAGAZINE** as published between the years 1850 and 1859, the period when hair work was promoted as the ladies drawing room pastime.

In addition to basic instructions and patterns an extensive catalog of hair jewelry and findings is presented with original prices as an excellent reference for the collector and historian. Unfortunately such findings are no longer available although the designs are clear enough for reproduction by a competant goldsmith.

TOOLS AND MATERIALS

MATERIALS

HAIR

The unique qualities of hair, particularly its wiry nature and ability to be set, make it the most desirable material for many of the patterns. Human or horse hair is still commercially available and should be experimented with. Horse hair was some times combined with human hair to give the finished work support. As a general rule, a finished piece of hair work will be about half the length of the starting strand. If hair strands are long enough, a double strand is preferable, i.e. long enough for two strands. In this case a bobbin would be attached to each end.

OTHER MATERIALS

As many of the hair designs rely on the unique characteristics of hair, substitute materials of similar qualities should be considered. Fine wire in copper, gold and silver can work in many of the patterns. Monofilament nylon, which can be dyed is available in a variety of weights can also be experimented with. When using wire, use several strands of the finest gauge as you would with hair. Do not wind the wire on the bobbins but use in manner and lengths as described for hair.

TOOLS

For tools, reference should be made to that available for working Kumi-Himo, which has gained much popularity in the last several years.

The essential tools are the *BOBBINS* which hold the working strands in tension, a *STAND* to support the work and maintain the position of the working strands, *MOLDS* to control the shape of the hollow braids and a *COUNTERBALANCE* to keep the work in position.

BOBBINS

Bobbins as used for lace making and tapestry weaving can be used for hair braiding techniques providing they are properly weighted. The weight of the bobbins will have a significant effect on the finished result and experimentation should be made with the different patterns and materials used.

A suggested bobbin is the *English Style* lace bobbin, These are slender and have a hole drilled near the bottom for attaching weights (beads) by means of a wire loop. This gives you the flexibility of adjusting the weight as best suited for the material/design being worked. The weights can be small lead fishing weights, curtain weights, washers or decorative beads. If other style bobbin are being used, holes can be drilled near the base to similarly hold weights. A good starting weight would be 1/2 to 3/4 oz per bobbin.

COUNTERBALANCE

The center or *COUNTERBALANCE* weight can be a simple muslin bag filled with sand or lead weights, again adjusted to the piece being worked. The weight of the counter balance should be approximately half the weight of all the bobbins.

THREAD

A starting or binding thread is required which is attached to the ends of the bundled strand of hairs. Linen is recommended in a size 60/2 for its strength and fineness.

STAND

The simplest form of stand can be a round cylindrical box such as a hat box or commercial ice-cream container. The top of the stand particularly the edge should be smooth. A small hole in the center must be made through which the working braid will pass. The edge should be sanded and sealed to insure the hair will not snag. Sealing wax placed around this edge will form a smooth hard surface which will not harm the fine hair.

MOLDS

Most hair braids are hollow and require a mold over which the braid is worked. For straight tubular braids a knitting needle or brass tube of appropriate size can be used. Molds, however of various shapes and designs can be made to create a variety of shapes such as beaded and tapered designs. Forms for this type can be made by wood turning. The molds must withstand the boiling process which is used to fix the worked shapes.

WORKING NOTES

In securing the thread to the bobbins use the half hitch method as diagrammed. This not only secures the thread to the bobbin, but it permits the thread to be shortened or extended without undoing the knot. If your thread is properly secured to the bobbin, the bobbin should hang without unwinding and yet should permit controlled release of the cord. A simple twist of the bobbin, in a direction opposite to that wound, while holding the attached cord in tension with the opposite hand, will unwind the cord.

All braids are a repeat of a series of motions of one or more bobbins. The bobbins are typically divided into groups and then the motions are by bobbins

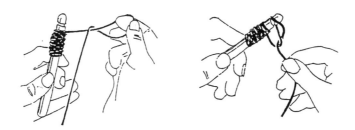

SECURING THREAD TO BOBBIN

within the group of between the groups. When the entire *described* sequence is complete you are ready to repeat the sequence. It will be noted that several braids are a combinations of alternating patterns. It is a simple matter to go from one pattern into another providing the number of groups is compatable. It is suggested that the stand be marked into sections, the number based on the pattern being worked. This can easily be done with small pieces of masking tape which can later be removed. The working sequences for projects in this book are characteristically shown by a single diagram with an explanation of the movements. We suggest that the diagrams and movements be studied prior to start of work with separate diagrams drawn and numbered for each motion. Each diagram should indicate the bobbins being moved and the position of the last moved bobbins (from the previous motion). As an example the braid from page 24 is drawn as suggested with each of the 8 movements shown by a separate diagram. The solid circles indicate the bobbin to be moved and the dotted circles indicate the moved bobbins. The arrows indicate starting and ending position and direction of movement.

The concept of combining the hair from loved ones can be very effective,

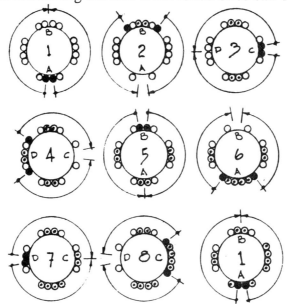

particularly if of a contrasting color. The groups of different color hair should be arranged symmetrically and symbolically noted on your working diagrams.

To fix the hair of the completed braid, immerse the work, with mold intact in boiling water and keep it there for 5-10 minutes. Dry thoroughly in a warm oven before withdrawing the mold.

REFERENCES

INDOR I VAMHUS SOCKEN, Uppsala 1966. Swedish Hair Braiding
KUMU HIMO, Jules & Kaethe Kliot. Illustrates kumi himo equipment and techniques as well as designs for a variety of braids.

SUPPLIES

LACIS, 2982 Adeline St., Berkeley, CA 94703
Books and related naterials for hair work, kumi-himo, lace making, embroidery and costume. Send $4.00 for catalog.

PREFACE.

The necessity for a comprehensive work, giving a full and detailed explanation of the Art of manufacturing Hair Work in all its various branches, has been so frequently urged upon the attention of the author, that, in compliance with an almost universal demand, he has concluded to publish a book which will clearly illustrate the Art of Hair Dressing, and making Hair Jewelry and Hair Work of every description. His perfect familiarity with the business—the result of many years' successful experience—renders him eminently competent to impart the fullest information upon the subject of which he treats, while the great consumption and rapidly increasing demand for every description of Hair Goods, will make this work he now presents to the public, one of particular interest to all classes. Heretofore the Art of making these goods has been zealously guarded by a few dealers, who have accumulated fortunes, and would still retain it a profound secret but for the publication of this book. This is the only descriptive volume ever published on Hair Work. It is an elaborate, carefully prepared book, containing over one thousand drawings, devices and diagrams, engraved at great expense to the publisher, and accompanied with the most comprehensive instructions. It not only reveals to the most ordinary comprehension the hitherto concealed mysteries of the Art, but will prove an indispensable adjunct to every lady's toilet table, as by its aid she will not only be able to dress her own hair in every variety of style, but make her own Hair Jewelry and articles of Hair Work, including Switches, Braids, Curls, Waterfalls, etc., assisted by a reference to plates of the most modern European and American styles.

For children, no art or accomplishment is more useful than the ability to make articles of tasteful ornament in Hair Work. This work will open to all such persons a path to agreeable and profitable occupation. Jewelry Dealers, from the clear instructions herein given, can manufacture any required pattern of Hair Jewelry, and add, without extra expense, a new and lucrative branch to their business.

Persons wishing to preserve, and weave into lasting mementoes, the hair of a deceased father, mother, sister, brother, or child, can also enjoy the inexpressible advantage and satisfaction of *knowing* that the material of their own handiwork is the actual hair of the "loved and gone."

No other work ever met with such an earnest demand as this treatise upon the art of Hair Braiding. It must certainly commend itself to the ladies of our country as invaluable. Even a hasty perusal will convince every one of its utility and worth. Translations in French and German are in progress.

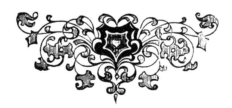

Synopsis of Human Hair.

IN placing before the public the only book ever published on the "Art of Hair Work," it is but due to the purchasers of it to say something in relation to the trade in Human Hair. It is not my intention, however, to enter into an extended detail and complete history, but simply give a few items that will serve to show what enormous strides have been taken, within the last few years, in this branch of business. It is a business that but few know anything about—at least in this country, for it is comparatively new here—but it is one that is very rapidly increasing, and is now almost doubling itself each year.

The larger quantity, in fact nearly the whole amount of hair retailed in this country is imported from Europe, where the dealing in human hair has been made an established and legitimate business for years, and a great deal of attention is paid to purchasing and preparing it for the market. Paris is the greatest market, for the sale of human hair, in the world; but the amount of superfluous hair used and worn throughout all Europe, could we give the figures, would seem incredible. The amount imported by the United States in the years 1859 and 1860 was not far from 150,000 or 200,000 pounds, which was valued at that time at from $800,000 to $1,000,000. Since that time it has been steadily increasing, and the amount imported last year may be set down at three times as much as during the years above mentioned. Paris also finds as great a sale for the article in Russia as in America, the shipments to each being about equal. Thus it will be seen, that if all the hair reserved in Europe for the home demand were added to that which is exported, the amount would be almost beyond conception; and yet, but about one-tenth part of the whole production ever leaves its native country.

It is mostly procured from the markets of France, Italy, Russia and Germany, and large quantities are obtained from Norway and Sweden.

The Norwegians were among the first to make ornaments of hair to be worn as jewelry; but, in a great measure, we are indebted to the French for the perfection to which the art has attained. Of the different varieties of hair, that which is obtained in France and Italy is by far the best, being of a much finer texture, even color, and of a more glossy appearance than that from other countries.

The principal requirement in hair, to make it valuable, is length; and after it is thrown upon the market it is all assorted—the long from the short—which is a task of extreme difficulty.

The prices of hair range all the way from $15 to $200 per pound, (a wide range, but certainly not too large,) and is rated according to hue, length and texture. The smallest price paid is for the short, coarse hair, of the poorest quality, and which can be used only for certain purposes. Hair of the ordinary colors ranges in price from $15 to $100 per pound, but that of gray and white from $100 to $200 per pound, and even then is not considered exorbitant. In fact, hair is worth any and all prices. We know of one dealer who had in his possession a very small quantity, weighing but a half pound, and measuring seventy inches, for which he was offered *four hundred dollars!* and, strange as it may appear, he refused to accept it. White hair is mostly obtained by being picked from the gray, and it not unfrequently happens that many hundred pounds have to be assorted before being able to secure one single pound of pure white. It is mainly used in the manufacture of wigs, and it frequently puzzles the dealer to prepare one for a customer that will exactly match; and this, with the scarcity of the article, causes the extraordinary price.

Hair is shipped in both a prepared and unprepared state. That which is prepared undergoes a process of washing, scouring and cleansing, which leaves it in the nicest possible state. All the oil, dirt and other unhealthy substances are completely separated from it, leaving it perfectly free from all unhealthy influences. That which is shipped in an unprepared, or raw state, is subjected to the same process of cleansing after its arrival, and it is so thorough that it is altogether impossible for anything except the hair to remain. It has frequently been examined with a microscope, which has proved in every case how successful the cleansing process had been, for it revealed nothing whatever of a foreign nature; and, in fact, after its extraordinary cleansing, it would be simply impossible.

After being fully prepared, it is then made into switches, curls, plaits, fronts, wigs, chignons, and not a small amount is used in the manufacture of hair jewelry, and such other articles as are worn for ornaments. The jewelry manufactured at this time is as durable as the all-gold jewelry, and is done in a style of surpassing neatness, thus rendering it beautiful, either as an ornament or memento. There are but very few places in the United States where hair jewelry is made; and as it is comparatively a new business, but few have learned it. It is surprising, however, to notice the many beautiful patterns and elegant designs into which it is transformed. There is nothing in the way of jewelry, or ornament of any description, but what is or may be made from human hair; and, after being gold-mounted, the contrast between them makes the hair jewelry preferable to the all-gold.

There are many strange incidents related of the human hair suddenly changing its color — many of which it is hard to believe — and the causes assigned are various. We are told of persons who, from excessive grief, found their hair had gradually changed from a dark brown to an almost perfect white; others, from the same cause, in the short space of one week discovered their hair plentifully streaked with gray, giving them the appearance, although young, of being quite old. Many have had their hair change on account of extreme fright; but we have now to give the first instance we have ever heard of its turning from white to that of any other color, except by the aid of dyes.

A Parisian, M. Stanislaus Martin, has published in the *Bulletin de Therapeutique* the curious case of a worker in metals who had wrought in copper only five months, and whose hair, which was lately white, is now of so decided a *green* that the man can not appear in the street without immediately becoming the object of general curiosity. He is perfectly well, his hair alone being affected by the copper, notwithstanding the precautions taken by him to protect it from the action of the metal. Chemical analysis shows that his hair contains a notable quantity of acetate of copper, and that it is to this circumstance that it owes its beautiful green color, which is most singular and remarkable.

The practice of wearing false hair, although it was not generally dealt in as traffic, has been in vogue many hundred years. The Greek and Roman ladies were, in olden times, as active in their toilet for the head as the fashionable ladies of the present day, and false hair was always brought into requisition, which was then obtained from the Germans, and they in turn from their slaves.

Powdering the hair, which is now the rage in all fashionable circles, is also an ancient practice, and was as much indulged in by the men as the women. History tells us that the consumption of hair powder by the soldiers of George II. was enormous. It was calculated, that inasmuch as the military force of England and the colonies was, including cavalry, infantry, militia and fensibles, 250,000, each man used a pound of flour a week, simply for powdering the hair. The quantity consumed in this way was 6,500 tons per annum; an amount sufficient to sustain 30,000 persons on bread. Gold and silver hair powder was also plentifully used, and at a time much earlier in the world's history than is generally supposed. Josephus relates that Solomon's horse-guards daily strewed their heads with gold-dust, which glittered in the sun; and there are similar instances of different personages recorded in the Bible.

The human hair seems to have been given us both for an ornament and covering—being susceptible of transformation into almost any desired shape, and apparently indispensable for covering and protecting the head. The ancient Greeks were very partial to long hair, considering it by far the more becoming; but the Egyptians regarded it as an incumbrance, shaved their heads, and substituted wigs. The ancients, generally speaking, strangely considered a fine head of hair so desirable, that it became sacred. They frequently dedicated it to the gods, on important occasions of marriage, victory, escape from death and danger, and the burial of friends. Different styles of wearing the hair were resorted to for denoting the various grades, or positions in life, of the people, some wearing it quite long, others short, and some dressing it in a peculiar manner,—each style, or length, being according to the condition, wealth or social standing of the wearer. Plucking it out, or neglecting it, was a token of affliction.

Hair contains a very small quantity of water, manganese, iron, and various salts of lime, which have been found by the various methods of analyzation, and it is owing to these properties that it is peculiarly indestructible. It has been found on mummies, more than twenty centuries old, in a perfect and unaltered state, and many instances are related, which are now admitted to be facts, of the hair continuing to grow, for a time, after death.

There has never before been a book written and published that was particularly dedicated to the subject of Hair, and as the field is a vast one, both as regards the importance of the subject and the information to be gained thereby, it is simply strange that no one has ever entered it. It has been too long neglected, and the increasing necessity for a treatise of this kind has been pressed upon the attention of the author, and induced the publication of this work, which will certainly meet the necessities of the age.

There is much else that might be said on this subject that would prove both interesting and instructive, but we prefer for the present to let it rest. We have endeavored, in preparing this book, both to instruct and amuse ; for, by following its instructions, it may be made to be profitable and highly remunerative, and in making articles, either for gifts, mementos, or otherwise, it will certainly be amusing and entertaining. We have given the instructions in a way that all may readily understand, and as the patterns are numerous, and the designs elegant, we think there can be nothing lacking to make the book all it claims to be.

Directions for New Beginners.

THE hair to be used in braiding should be combed perfectly straight, and tied with a string at the roots, to prevent wasting. Then count the number of hairs for a strand, and pull it out from the tips, dip it in water, and draw it between the thumb and finger to make it lie smoothly. Then tie a solid single knot at one end, the same as you would with a sewing thread.

THE BOBBIN.

To prepare the bobbin for the hair, wind it with white thread, as shown in the plate, and fasten it with a slip-knot over the knob, leaving an end of some three inches, with a solid knot tied at the end of it. To adjust the hair to the bobbins, take the prepared strands of hair and tie the knotted ends in a square knot to the ends of the strings on the bobbins. When each strand is thus prepared and tied to the bobbin strings, place them even, and tie the ends with a string to prevent their slipping.

See cut of bobbins on another page.

HOW TO PLACE THEM ON THE TABLE-COVER FOR BRAIDING.

Place the strands across the table-cover, over the numbers, as shown in the diagram, and fasten a weight to the end of them, under the table, through the center of the cover; then tie the mold, or form to be braided, around in the center, and you are ready for braiding.

For further reference, see plate of table, with explanations.

Braiding Table.

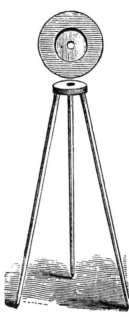

No. 1.

The Table-cover, as shown in diagram No. 1, represents the under side of the cover, showing the rim that fits over the cap, allowing the cover to revolve, for the convenience of the braider.   The cavity through the cover and cap allows the braid, with the weight attached, to pass through as fast as braided.

For reference, see Braiding Table complete, with bobbins and weights attached, on page 18 .

Braiding Table.

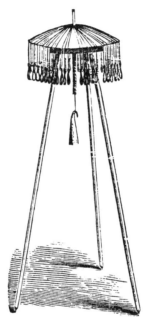

No. 2.

The above cut represents Braiding Table No. 2, complete, showing the strands over the cover, with bobbins attached; also, the weight attached to the braid, showing the manner of its passing through the table.

Wood Braiding Bobbins.

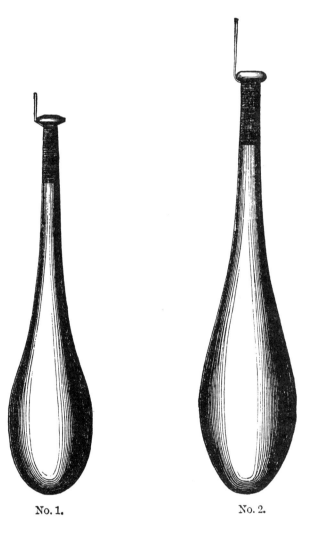

No. 1.   No. 2.

The above cut shows the Wood Bobbins, for fine open work or tight braids. No. 1 is used for braiding any pattern of from one to four hairs in a strand. No. 2 is used for braiding any pattern of from five to twenty hairs in a strand. To prepare the bobbins for use, see explanations on page 16.

Lead Bobbins.

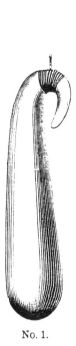

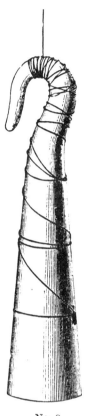

No. 1.   No. 2.

The above cuts show the size and shape of the Lead Bobbins. The No. 1 size is used for braiding rings and chains that have but few hairs in a strand—from twenty to forty. No. 2 is used for braiding chains that have from forty to one hundred hairs in a strand. Either size will answer for any pattern of chain or ring, but to vary the size of the bobbin according to the number of hairs in a strand, gives it a nicer finish. To prepare the bobbin, wind it with thread, as shown in the cut, leaving the thread some three inches long, with a solid knot tied at the end.

Lead Weight.

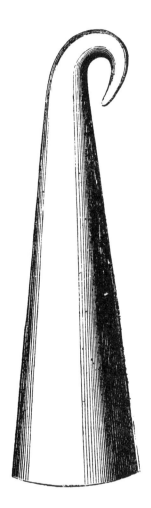

The above cut shows the weight used for drawing the work through the center of the table as fast as braided, and to balance the bobbins. Attention should be given to have the weight balance the bobbins properly, as too great a weight will make the braid loose, or too light a weight will leave it rough. Use any number of weights required to balance the bobbins.

Forms for Braiding Over.

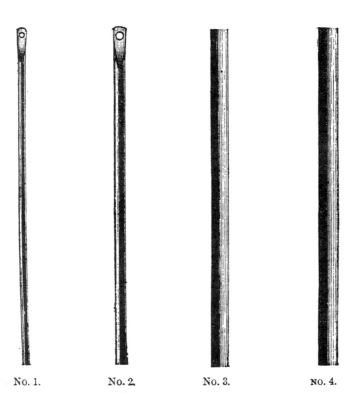

No. 1.   No. 2.   No. 3.   NO. 4.

The above cuts are made of wire and wood, for braiding over. The Nos. 1 and 2 are for braiding chains over—the No. 1 for small chains and the No 2 for large sizes.   No. 3 is used for braiding tight or open work braids, of from thirty to forty strands.   No. 4 is used for the same braids, with from forty to sixty strands in a braid.   The mold may be made any length to accommodate the work.

Forms for Braiding Over.

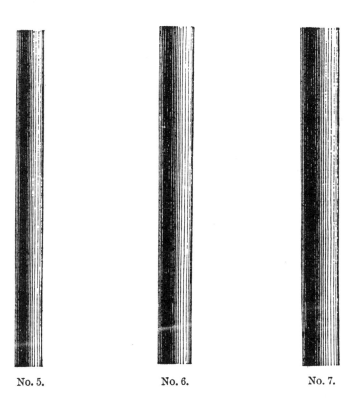

No. 5.　　　　　　No. 6.　　　　　　No. 7.

The above cuts show the size of forms used for tight or open work braids. The No. 5 is used for braids of from sixty to eighty strands, No. 6 of from eighty to one hundred, and No. 7 from one hundred to one hundred and twenty, according to the fineness of the braid.

INTRODUCTORY REMARKS

In this book of instruction I have introduced for practice the easiest braids first—which are chain braids. The first pattern, found on page 9, is a very easy and handsome one, and should be practiced to perfection before trying any other, as it will enable the beginner to execute all others after the first is perfected: A new beginner should be particular to place the strands correctly upon the table, and mark the cover with precision, after the manner shown in the diagram. I have, by the introduction of plates, diagrams, and explanatory remarks, made comprehensive and simple the execution of all the braids herein contained. The novice should first give special attention to preparing the hair for braiding, the adjustment of it to the bobbins, weights, molds, etc., of which plates and full explanations are to be found elsewhere in this book. I wish to impress upon the mind of the worker, that every change made with the strands changes the numbers of them to correspond with the numbers on the table. For example: lift No. 1 over No. 2, which would make No. 1 No. 2, and No. 2 No. 1, etc.

Square Chain Braid.

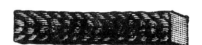

TAKE sixteen strands, eighty hairs in a strand, and place on table like pattern. Commence at A, take Nos. 1—one in each hand—lift them over the table, one on each side of the mold, and lay them between Nos. 1 at B, and bring back the Nos. 2 from B, one on each side of the mold, and lay them between Nos. 2 at A; then go to C, lift Nos. 1 over between Nos. 1 at D, passing one strand each side of the 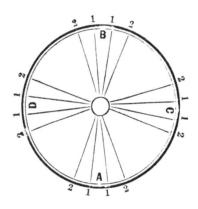 mold, and bring back Nos. 2 from D, and lay between Nos. 2 at C. Then go to B and braid the same, then to D, and so on around to the right, until the braid is finished.

Braid this over a mold, made of small wire, with a hole in one end like the eye of a needle, so as to draw a small cord in the place of the wire. When you have it braided, take off the weights, tie the ends fast on the wire, and push the braid tight together; then boil in water about ten minutes, and take it out and put in an oven as hot as it will bear without burning, until quite dry; then slip it off the wire on to the cord, sew the ends of the braid so it will not slip, and put a little shellac on the end to keep it fast. If you want it elastic, use elastic cord. To vary the size of the braid, vary the number of hairs in a strand.

Reverse Chain Braid.

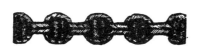

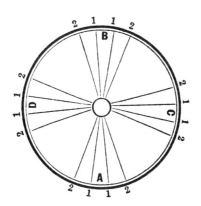

TAKE sixteen strands, and place on table like pattern. Commence at A, with sixty hairs in a strand. Take Nos. 2, lift over table to B, lay them in between Nos. 1 at B, and bring back Nos. 2 from B, and lay in between Nos. 1 at A. Then walk around table to C; take Nos. 1 and lift over table and lay them in between Nos. 1 at D, and bring back Nos. 1 from D to C; then take Nos. 2 at C, lift over table and lay them inside of Nos. 2 at D, and bring back Nos. 2 from D to C. After braiding several times round to suit your taste, say five, reverse the braid by commencing at C, and braiding as you did at A, by taking Nos. 2 at C, lift over table to D, and lay them in between Nos. 1 at D, and bring back Nos. 2 from D, and lay in between Nos. 1 at C. Then go to A, and take Nos. 1, lift over table and lay in between Nos. 1 at B, and bring back Nos. 1 from B to A; then take Nos. 2 at A, lift over table and lay in between Nos. 2 at B, and fetch back Nos. 2 from B to A; then commence' at C again, and braid five times. Then commence at A as you did at first, reversing it every time you braid it five times through. Braid it over a small wire, tie the ends on the wire, boil and dry the same as chain on page nine, only you need not press the braid together on the wire.

Sixteen Twist Chain.

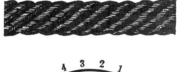

TAKE sixteen strands, eighty hairs in a strand, and place on table like pattern. Commence at A and B; take No. 1 at A in right hand, and No. 1 at B in left hand, and swing them around the table to the right, changing places with them. Take Nos. 1 at C and D and change as at A and B. Then go to B and take Nos. 2 at B and A, and change them by taking No. 2 at B in right hand and No. 2 at

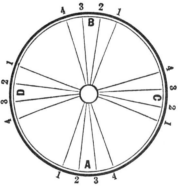

A in left hand, and swing them around table to the right as before, changing places with them. Then go around the table to D, and take Nos. 2 at D and C, and change places as before. Then take Nos. 3 at A and B, and change as before; then take Nos. 3 at C and D, and change places with them. Then take Nos. 4 at B and A, and change as before. Then take Nos. 4 at D and C, and change as before. Then commence at A, as at first, repeating until the braid is finished.

Striped Snake Chain Braid.

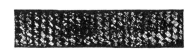

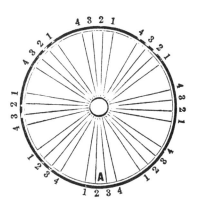

AKE thirty-two strands, with twelve hairs in a strand, or any number that can be divided by four, and sixty strands for usual size, and place them on table like pattern. Have every alternate two strands of black hair, and the others of light hair. Commence at A, taking two strands of light hair in left hand, Nos. 1 and 2, and take two strands of black hair in right hand, Nos. 3 and 4, and cross No. 2 (light) over No. 3 (dark), then No. 1 (light) under No. 3 (dark), then No. 4 (dark) over Nos. 1 and 2 (light); so on around the table to the right until you get to A; then commence and work back to the left, by taking light hair in left hand and dark hair in right hand, as before, and put No. 3 (dark) over No. 2 (light), and No. 4 (dark) under No. 2 (light), and No. 1 (light) over Nos. 3 and 4 (dark); so on around the table till you get to A; then commence as at first, so on, braiding first one way round the table, then the other, till you have the chain completed.

Braid it over wood, or brass wire, the size and length you wish your chain. When braided, take off your weights, tie the ends fast and boil and dry, then take out the mold and put a cord through with some cotton wrapped around it so it will be soft and pliable. This is called the STRIPED SNAKE BRAID, and can be braided all of one color if desired.

Cable Chain Braid.

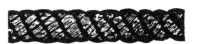

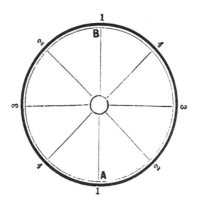

TAKE any number of strands that can be divided by two, with eighty hairs in a strand, twenty strands for usual size, and place them on table like pattern. Commencing, take No. 1 at A in right hand and No. 1 at B in left hand, and swing around the table to the right, and lay the one in right hand at No. 1 at B and the one in left hand at No. 1 at A; then bring back No. 2 at B with right hand and No. 2 at A in left hand, and swing round table to the left; then take No. 3, and swing to the right; then No. 4, and swing to the left; so on round, first to the right, then to the left, with every number of the strands, till you get to No. 1; then commence as at first, and so on till the chain is as long as required.

Braid this over a small wire, with a hole in one end like the eye of a needle, so as to draw a small cord in the place of the wire. When you have it braided, take off your weights, tie the ends fast on the wire, and push the braid together; then boil in water about ten minutes; then take it out and put it in an oven as hot as it will bear without burning, until it is quite dry; then take it out and slip it off the wire on to the cord, sew the ends of the braid so it will not slip on the cord, and put a little shellac on the end to keep it fast. If you want it elastic, use elastic cord. To vary the size of the braid, vary the number of hairs in a strand.

Snake Chain Braid.

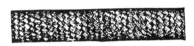

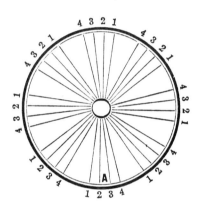

TAKE thirty-two strands, or any number that can be divided by four, twelve hairs in a strand, and sixty strands for usual size; place them on table like pattern. Commence at A, lift No. 2 in your right hand, and put your left under your right hand, and take up No. 3 and bring it back of No. 1, and lay them both down; then take up No. 4 and lay it between Nos. 1 and 2; then take the next four to the right, and so on till you get around the table; then commence and braid back around the table to the left, but reverse the braid by braiding it this way: Lift No. 3 with your left hand, pass your right under and take No. 2, and bring it back over No. 4, and lay them both down; then take No. 1 and lift it over in between Nos. 3 and 4, and so on till you get around the table. Then commence as at first, braid one way, then the other, till you have it as long as required.

Braid it over wood, or brass wire, the size and length you wish your chain. When braided, take off your weights, tie the ends fast and boil and dry; then take out the mold and put a cord through, with some cotton wrapped around it so that it will be soft and pliable. This is called the SNAKE CHAIN BRAID.

Eight-Square Chain Braid.

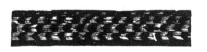

AKE sixteen strands, eighty hairs in a strand, and place them on table like pattern. Commence at A: take Nos. 1 strands, lift across the table and lay down inside of Nos. 1 at B, and bring back Nos. 1 from B to A; then lift Nos. 2 at A over inside of Nos. 2 at B, and bring back Nos. 2 from B to A; then lift Nos. 3 from A to B, and bring back Nos. 3 from B to A; then lift

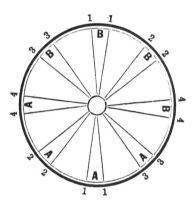

Nos. 4 from A to B, and bring back Nos. 4 from B to A; then commence at Nos. 1 again, and repeat until the chain is completed.

Braid this over a small wire, with a hole in one end like the eye of a needle, so as to draw a small cord in the place of the wire. When you have it braided, take off your weights, tie the ends fast on the wire, and push the braid together; then boil in water about ten minutes; then take it out and put it in an oven as hot as it will bear without burning, until it is quite dry; then take it out and slip it off the wire on to the cord, sew the ends of the braid so it will not slip on the cord, and put a little shellac on the end to keep it fast. If you want it elastic, use elastic cord. To vary the size of the braid, vary the number of hairs in a strand.

Half Twist Chain Braid.

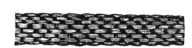

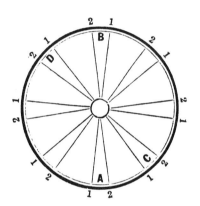

TAKE sixteen strands, or any number that can be divided by two, usually eighty hairs in a strand. Commence at A and B: take No. 1 at A in right hand and No. 1 at B in left hand, and swing them around table to the right, and lay the one in right hand down at B, across over No. 2, and the one in left hand lay down across over No. 2 at A; then go to C and D, and change No. 1 as before at A and B; then go to the next two strands, and change as before; so on around the table, taking the next two each time, until the chain is completed.

Braid this over a small wire, with a hole in one end like the eye of a needle, so as to draw a small cord in the place of the wire. When you have it braided, take off your weights, tie the ends fast on the wire, and push the braid together; then boil in water about ten minutes; then take it out and put it in an oven as hot as it will bear without burning, until it is quite dry; then take it out and slip it off the wire on to the cord, sew the ends of the braid so it will not slip on the cord, and put a little shellac on the end to keep it fast. If you want it elastic, use elastic cord. To vary the size of the braid, vary the number of hairs in a strand.

Square Chain Braid.

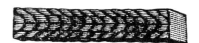

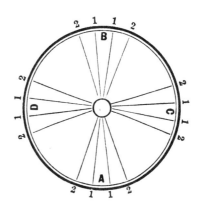

TAKE sixteen strands, eighty hairs in a strand, and place on table like pattern. Commence at A, lift Nos. 1 across table and lay in between Nos. 1 at B, and bring back Nos. 1 from B to A; then go to C, take Nos. 1 and lift across table and lay in between Nos. 1 at D, and bring back Nos. 1 from D to C; then go to A, take Nos. 2 and lift across inside of Nos. 2 at B, and bring back Nos. 2 from B to A; then go to C, lift Nos. 2 across inside of Nos. 2 at D, and bring back Nos. 2 from D to C; then go to A, and commence as at first, and repeat until it is the required length.

Braid this over a small wire, with a hole in one end like the eye of a needle, so as to draw a small cord in the place of the wire. When you have it braided, take off your weights, tie the ends fast on the wire, and push the braid close together; then boil in water about ten minutes, and take it out and put it in an oven as hot as it will bear without burning, until it is quite dry; then take it out and slip it off the wire on to the cord, sew the ends of the braid so it will not slip, and put a little shellac on the ends to keep it fast. If you want it elastic, use elastic cord. To vary the size of the braid, vary the number of hairs in a strand.

Cable Twist Chain Braid.

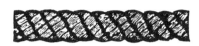

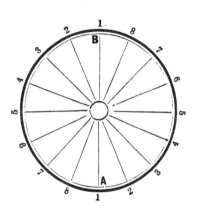

TAKE sixteen strands, eighty hairs in a strand, and place them on table like pattern. Commence at A and B, with Nos. 1, passing them around table to the right, and leave No. 1 from A at B and No. 1 from B at A; then take Nos. 7 at A and B, and pass around table to right, and leave the one from A at B and the one from B at A; then take Nos. 2 at A and B, changing places with them; then take Nos. 8, and change as before; then take Nos. 3 at A and B, and change them as before; then take Nos. 1 at A and B, and change as at first; then take Nos. 4, and change as before; then take Nos. 2, and change as before; then take Nos. 5, and change as before; so on until the braid is finished, all the time taking the third strand to the right, or forward, and the second one to the left, or backward.

Braid this over a small wire, with a hole in one end like the eye of a needle, so as to draw a small cord in the place of the wire. When you have it braided, take off your weights, tie the ends fast on the wire, and push the braid together; then boil in water about ten minutes; then take it out and put it in an oven as hot as it will bear without burning, until it is quite dry; then take it out and slip it off the wire on to the cord, sew the ends of the braid so it will not slip on the cord, and put a little shellac on the end to keep it fast. If you want it elastic, use elastic cord. To vary the size of the braid, vary the number of hairs in a strand.

Twist Chain Braid.

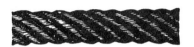

AKE eighteen strands, eighty hairs in a strand, and place them on table like pattern. Commence at A and B: take Nos. 1, and swing around table to the right, and place the No. 1 from A over the Nos. 2 and 3 at B, and the No. 1 from B over the Nos. 2 and 3 at A; then go to C and D, take the Nos. 1 and change the same; then go to E and F, and change the same; then

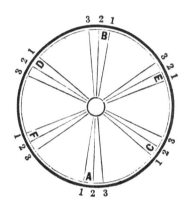

go to B and A, and change as at first, (all the time taking the Nos. 1 and swinging to the right, for when you lay them over the Nos. 2 and 3 it makes them Nos. 3, and makes Nos. 2 Nos. 1,) and so on, until the chain is finished.

Braid this over a small wire, with a hole in one end like the eye of a needle, so as to draw a small cord in the place of the wire. When you have it braided, take off your weights, tie the ends fast on the wire, and push the braid together; then boil in water about ten minutes; then take it out and put it in an oven as hot as it will bear without burning, until it is quite dry; then take it out and slip it off the wire on to the cord, sew the ends of the braid so it will not slip on the cord, and put a little shellac on the end to keep it fast. If you want it elastic, use elastic cord. To vary the size of the braid, vary the number of hairs in a strand.

Twist Chain Braid.

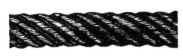

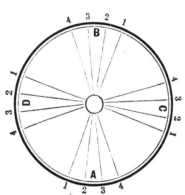

TAKE sixteen strands, eighty hairs in a strand, and place them on table like pattern. Commence at A and B: take No. 1 at A in right hand and No. 1 at B in left hand, and swing them around the table to the right, and lay the one in the right hand down at B, over across Nos. 2, 3 and 4, and the one in the left hand at A, over across Nos. 2, 3 and 4; then go to C, and take Nos. 1 at C and D, and change as before at A and B; then go to B, and take Nos. 1 at B and A and change them, by taking No. 1 at B in right hand and No. 1 at A in left hand, and swing them round the table to the right as before, laying them across over Nos. 2, 3 and 4; so on, braiding around the table to the right, until you have it the required length.

Braid this over a small wire, with a hole in one end like the eye of a needle, so as to draw a small cord in the place of the wire. When you have it braided, take off your weights, tie the ends fast on the wire, and push the braid close together; then boil in water about ten minutes, and take it out and put it in an oven as hot as it will bear without burning, until it is quite dry; then take it out and slip it off the wire on to the cord, sew the ends of the braid so it will not slip on the cord, and put a little shellac on the ends to keep it fast. If you want it elastic, use elastic cord. To vary the size of the braid, vary the number of hairs in a strand.

Rib Chain Braid.

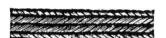

AKE sixteen strands, eighty hairs in a strand, and place them on table like pattern. Commence at A : take Nos. 2, and lift over across table outside of Nos. 2 at B, and bring back Nos. 1 from B to A outside of Nos. 1 at A; then take Nos. 1 at C, and cross over inside of Nos. 1 at D, and bring back Nos. 2 from D inside of Nos. 2 at C; then go back to A, and braid as before, so on repeating until it is finished.

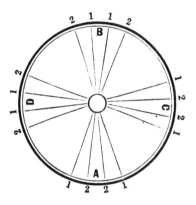

Braid this over a small wire, with a hole in one end like the eye of a needle, so as to draw a small cord in the place of the wire. When you have it braided, take off your weights, tie the ends fast on the wire, and push the braid together on the wire; then boil in water about ten minutes; then take it out, and put in an oven as hot as it will bear without burning, until it is quite dry; then take it out, and slip it off the wire on to the cord, and sew the ends of the braid so it will not slip on the cord, and put a little shellac on the end to keep it fast. If you want it elastic, use elastic cord. To vary the size of the braid, vary the number of hairs in a strand.

Twist Chain Braid.

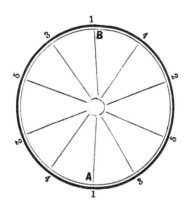

TAKE ten strands, with eighty hairs in a strand, and place them on table like pattern. Commence at A and B: Take Nos. 1 and swing them around the table to the right, and leave the No. 1 from A at B, and the No. 1 from B at A; then take Nos. 2 and swing them around the table to the right and change places with each other; then take Nos. 3 and change places as before; then take Nos. 4 and change places as before; then take Nos. 5 and change places as before; then commence at Nos. 1 and repeat until the braid is finished.

Braid this over a small wire, with a hole in one end like the eye of a needle, so as to draw a small cord in the place of the wire. When you have it braided, take off your weights, tie the ends fast on the wire, and push the braid together; then boil in water about ten minutes; then take it out and put it in an oven as hot as it will bear without burning, until it is quite dry; then take it out and slip it off the wire on to the cord, sew the ends of the braid so it will not slip on the cord, and put a little shellac on the end to keep it fast. If you want it elastic, use elastic cord. To vary the size of the braid, vary the number of hairs in a strand.

Half Twist Chain Braid.

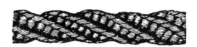

AKE sixteen strands, seventy-five hairs in a strand, and place on table like pattern. Commence at A: take Nos. 1 and 2, lift across the table to B, and lay No. 1 outside of No. 4, and lay No. 2 between Nos. 1 and 2, and bring back Nos. 1 and 2 from B to A, and lay No. 1 outside of No. 4 and No. 2 outside of No. 1 at A; then go to C, and take Nos. 1 and 2, lift over table

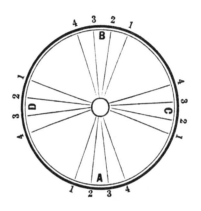

to D, and lay No. 1 outside of No. 4, and lay No. 2 between Nos. 1 and 2, and bring back Nos. 1 and 2 from C, and lay No. 1 outside of No. 4 and No. 2 outside of No. 1 at C; then go to B, and change the same, and so on around the table to the right until the braid is finished.

Braid this over a small wire, with a hole in one end like the eye of a needle, so as to draw a small cord in the place of the wire. When you have it braided, take off your weights, tie the ends fast on the wire, and push the braid together on the wire; then boil in water about ten minutes; then take it out, and put in an oven as hot as it will bear without burning, until it is quite dry; then take it out, and slip it off the wire on to the cord, and sew the ends of the braid so it will not slip on the cord, and put a little shellac on the end to keep it fast. If you want it elastic, use elastic cord. To vary the size of the braid, vary the number of hairs in a strand.

Cable Chain Braid.

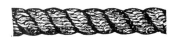

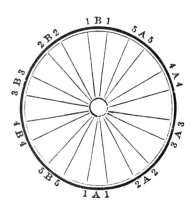

TAKE twenty strands, seventy-five hairs in a strand, and place them on table like pattern. Commence at A: lift Nos. 1 over across the table inside of Nos. 1 at B, and bring back Nos. 1 from B to A; then take Nos. 2 at A, cross over and lay them between Nos. 2 at B, and carry back Nos. 2 from B to A; then take Nos. 3 at A, cross over inside of Nos. 3 at B, and bring back Nos. 3 from B to A; then take Nos. 4 at A and cross over inside of Nos. 4 at B, and bring back Nos. 4 from B to A; then take Nos. 5 at A, cross over inside of Nos. 5 at B, and bring back Nos. 5 from B to A; then take Nos. 1 at B, cross over inside of Nos. 1 at A, and bring back Nos. 1 from A to B; then take Nos. 2 at B and cross over inside of Nos. 2 at A, and bring back Nos. 2 from A to B; then take Nos. 3, and so on around the table to the right, until the braid is finished, all the time taking the next two.

Braid this over a small wire, with a hole in one end like the eye of a needle, so as to draw a small cord in the place of the wire. When you have it braided, take off your weights, tie the ends fast on the wire, and push the braid together; then boil in water about ten minutes; then take it out and put it in an oven as hot as it will bear without burning, until it is quite dry; then take it out and slip it off the wire on to the cord, sew the ends of the braid so it will not slip on the cord, and put a little shellac on the end to keep it fast. If you want it elastic, use elastic cord. To vary the size of the braid, vary the number of hairs in a strand.

Sixteen Square Chain Braid.

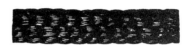

TAKE thirty-two strands, fifty hairs in a strand, and place on table like pattern. Commence at A, lift Nos. 1 across inside of Nos. 1 at B, and bring back Nos. 1 from B to A; then change at C and D, E and F, and G and H the same; then go to A, lift Nos. 2 across in place of Nos. 2 at B, and bring back Nos. 2 from B to A; then change at C and D, E and F, and G and H the same. Then you are through the braid, ready to commence at A, as at first, repeating the changes until the braid is finished.

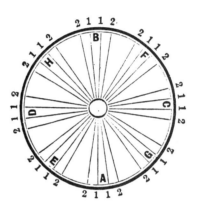

Braid this over a small wire, with a hole in one end like the eye of a needle, so as to draw a small cord in the place of the wire. When you have it braided, take off your weights, tie the ends fast on the wire, and push the braid close together; then boil in water about ten minutes, and take it out and put it in an oven as hot as it will bear without burning, until it is quite dry; then take it out and slip it off the wire on to the cord, sew the ends of the braid so it will not slip, and put a little shellac on the ends to keep it fast. If you want it elastic, use elastic cord. To vary the size of the braid, vary the number of hairs in a strand.

German Twist Chain Braid.

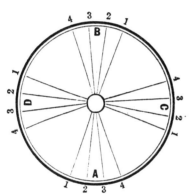

AKE sixteen strands, eighty hairs in a strand, and place them on table like pattern. Commence at A and B: take No. 1 at A in right hand and No. 1 at B in left hand, and swing them around to the right, and change places with them; then take No. 1 at C in right hand and No. 1 at D in left hand, and swing around table to the right, and change places as before; then take No. 2 at B in right hand and No. 2 at A in left hand, and swing to the right and change as before; then take No. 2 at D in right hand and No. 2 at C in left hand, and swing to the right and change as before; then take No. 3 at A in right hand and No. 3 at B in left hand, and change as before; then take No. 3 at C in right hand and No. 3 at D in left hand, and change as before; then take No. 4 at B in right hand and No. 4 at A in left hand, and change as before; then take No. 4 at D in right hand and No. 4 at C in left hand, and change as before. Then commence at A, as at first, and repeat till the braid is finished.

For further directions see page 9.

Fancy Square Chain Braid.

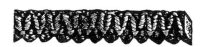

TAKE twenty-four strands, seventy hairs in a strand, and place on table like pattern. Commence at A: change Nos. 1 at A across inside of Nos. 1 at B, and bring back Nos. 1 from B to A; then go to C, change Nos. 1 across inside of Nos. 1 at D, and bring back Nos. 1 from D to C; then take No. 1 at E in right hand and No. 1 at F in left hand, lift across table in place of Nos. 1 at G and H,

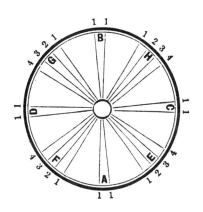

and bring back Nos. 1 from G and H to F and E; then take Nos. 2 at E and F, and change across to G and H, and lay in place of Nos. 2, and bring back Nos. 2 from G and H to F and E; then take Nos. 3, and change across to G and H as before; then take Nos. 4 at F and E, and change across to G and H as before; then go to C, and change the Nos. 1 across to D, and bring the Nos. 1 from D to C; then go to A, and change the Nos. 1 across to B, and bring back Nos. 1 from B to A; then go to E and H, take No. 4 at H in right hand, and No. 4 at E in left hand, and lift across in place of Nos. 4 at F and G, and bring back Nos. 4 from F and G to E and H; then take Nos. 3 at E and H, and change across in place of Nos. 3 at F and G, and bring back Nos. 3 from F and G to E and H; then take Nos. 2 at E and H, and change across in place of Nos. 2 at F and G, and bring back Nos. 2 from F and G to E and H; then take Nos. 1 at E and H, and change across in place of Nos. 1 at F and G, and bring back Nos. 1 from F and G to E and H; then go to A, and commence as at first, and repeat till the chain is finished.

For further directions, see page 9.

Fancy Square Chain Braid.

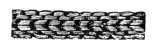

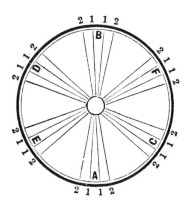

TAKE twenty-four strands, with seventy hairs in a strand, and place on table like pattern. Commence at A: lift Nos. 1 across inside of Nos. 1 at B, and bring back Nos. 1 from B to A; then change Nos. 1 at C and D the same; then change Nos. 1 at E and F the same; then go to A, lift Nos. 2 across to B, and bring back Nos. 2 from B to A; then change Nos. 2 at C and D the same; then change Nos. 2 at E and F the same, and you are through the braid, ready to commence at A, as at first.

Braid this over a small wire, with a hole in one end like the eye of a needle, so as to draw a small cord in the place of the wire. When you have it braided, take off your weights, tie the ends fast on the wire, and push the braid together; then boil in water about ten minutes; then take it out and put it in an oven as hot as it will bear without burning, until it is quite dry; then take it out and slip it off the wire on to the cord, sew the ends of the braid so it will not slip on the cord, and put a little shellac on the end to keep it fast. If you want it elastic, use elastic cord. To vary the size of the braid, vary the number of hairs in a strand.

Square Chain Braid.

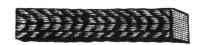

AKE sixteen strands, eighty hairs in a strand, and place on table like pattern. Commence at A: change the Nos. 1 across inside of Nos. 1 at B, and bring back Nos. 1 from B to A; then take Nos. 2 at A, change over in place of Nos. 2 at B, and bring back Nos. 2 from B to A; then go to C, and change the Nos. 1 from C to D, and bring back Nos. 1 from D to C; then take Nos. 2 at C, 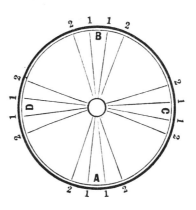 and change over in place of Nos. 2 at D, and bring back Nos. 2 from D to C; then go to A, and begin as at first, repeating until the braid is finished.

Braid this over a small wire, with a hole in one end like the eye of a needle, so as to draw a small cord in the place of the wire. When you have it braided, take off your weights, tie the ends fast on the wire, and push the braid close together; then boil in water about ten minutes, and take it out and put it in an oven as hot as it will bear without burning, until it is quite dry; then take it out and slip it off the wire on to the cord, sew the ends of the braid so it will not slip on the cord, and put a little shellac on the ends to keep it fast. If you want it elastic, use elastic cord. To vary the size of the braid, vary the number of hairs in a strand.

Fancy Twist Chain Braid.

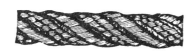

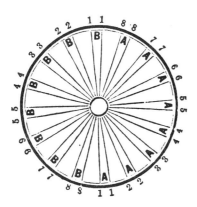

TAKE thirty-two strands, fifty hairs in a strand, and place them on table like pattern. Change Nos. 1 at A across inside of Nos. 1 at B, and bring back Nos. 1 from B to A; then change in the same way, successively, the Nos. 3, 5, 2, 4, 6, 3, 5, 7, 4, 6, 8, 5, 7, 1, 6, 8, 2, 7, 1, 3, 8, 2, 4. Then you are through, ready to commence as at first.

Braid this over a small wire, with a hole in one end like the eye of a needle, so as to draw a small cord in the place of the wire. When you have it braided, take off your weights, tie the ends fast on the wire, and push the braid together; then boil in water about ten minutes; then take it out and put it in an oven as hot as it will bear without burning, until it is quite dry; then take it out and slip it off the wire on to the cord, sew the ends of the braid so it will not slip on the cord, and put a little shellac on the end to keep it fast. If you want it elastic, use elastic cord. To vary the size of the braid, vary the number of hairs in a strand.

Fancy Twist Chain Braid.

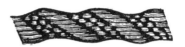

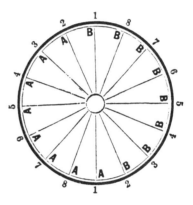

AKE sixteen strands, eighty hairs in a strand, and place them on table like pattern. Commence at A and B: take No. 1 at A in left hand and No. 1 at B in right hand, swing around table to the left, and change places with them; then take No. 7 at B in right hand and No. 7 at A in left hand, and swing around the table to the right, and change places with them; then take No. 5 at A in right hand and No. 5 at B in left hand, and swing around the table to the left, and change places as before; then take No. 8 at A in right hand and No. 8 at B in left hand, and swing around the table to the left, and change as before; then take No. 6 at A in left hand and No. 6 at B in right hand, and swing around table to the right, and change as before; then take No. 4 at A in right hand and No. 4 at B in left hand, and swing around table to the left, and change as before; then take No. 7 at A in right hand and No. 7 at B in left hand, swing around table to the left, and change as before; then take No. 5 at A in left hand and No. 5 at B in right hand, swing around table to the right, and change as before; then take No. 3 at A in right hand and No. 3 at B in left hand, and swing around table to the left, and change as before; then take No. 6 at A in right hand and No. 6 at B in left hand, and swing around table to the left, and change as before; then take No. 4 at A in left hand and No. 4 at B in right hand, and swing around table to the right, and change as before; then take No. 2 at A in right hand· and No. 2 at B in left hand, and swing around table to the left, and change as before; then take No. 5 at A in right hand and No. 5 at B in left hand, and swing around table to the left, and change as before; then take No. 3 at A in left hand and No. 3 at B in right hand, and swing around table to the right, and change as before; then commence at A, as at first.

Braid this over a small wire, with a hole in one end like the eye of a needle, so as to draw a small cord in the place of the wire. When you have it braided, take off your weights, tie the ends fast on the wire, and push the braid together; then boil in water about ten minutes; then take it out and put it in an oven as hot as it will bear without burning, until it is quite dry; then take it out and slip it off the wire on to the cord, sew the ends of the braid so it will not slip on the cord, and put a little shellac on the end to keep it fast. If you want it elastic, use elastic cord. To vary the size of the braid, vary the number of hairs in a strand.

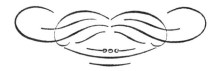

Double Twist Chain Braid.

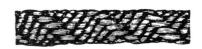

AKE eighteen strands, eighty hairs in a strand, and place them on table like pattern. Commence at A and B: take No. 1 at A in right hand and No. 1 at B in left hand, and swing them around the table to the right, and change places with them; then change the Nos. 8, 6 and 4 the same way; then count back five to the left (not counting the one last braided), bringing you to

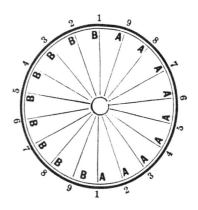

No. 9—swing as before to the right, and change places; then change the Nos. 7, 5 and 3 the same way; then count back five, bringing you to No. 8—change the same; and so on, first counting two forward and change three times, and then count five back and change the same; so on until the braid is finished.

Braid this over a small wire, with a hole in one end like the eye of a needle, so as to draw a small cord in the place of the wire. When you have it braided, take off your weights, tie the ends fast on the wire, and push the braid together; then boil in water about ten minutes; then take it out and put it in an oven as hot as it will bear without burning, until it is quite dry; then take it out and slip it off the wire on to the cord, sew the ends of the braid so it will not slip on the cord, and put a little shellac on the end to keep it fast. If you want it elastic, use elastic cord. To vary the size of the braid, vary the number of hairs in a strand.

Fancy Cable Chain Braid.

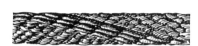

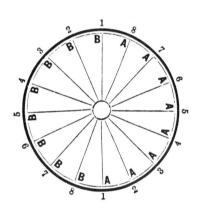

TAKE sixteen strands, eighty hairs in a strand, and place them on table like pattern. Commence at A and B: take No. 1 at A in right hand and No. 1 at B in left hand, and swing them around to the left and change places with them; then take, successively, Nos. 3, 5, 2, 4, 6, 3, 5, 7, 4, 6, 8, and change the same; then commence as at first with No. 1, so on repeating until the braid is finished.

Braid this over a small wire, with a hole in one end like the eye of a needle, so as to draw a small cord in the place of the wire. When you have it braided, take off your weights, tie the ends fast on the wire, and push the braid together; then boil in water about ten minutes; then take it out and put it in an oven as hot as it will bear without burning, until it is quite dry; then take it out and slip it off the wire on to the cord, sew the ends of the braid so it will not slip on the cord, and put a little shellac on the end to keep it fast. If you want it elastic, use elastic cord. To vary the size of the braid, vary the number of hairs in a strand.

Half Square Chain Braid.

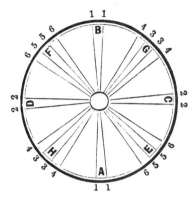

TAKE twenty-four strands, seventy hairs in a strand, and place on table like pattern. Commence at A: take Nos. 1, and lay them in the place of Nos. 1 at B, and bring back Nos. 1 from B to A; then take Nos. 2 at C, and lay in the place of Nos. 2 at D, and bring back Nos. 2 from D to C; then take the Nos. 3 from H and lay between the Nos. 3 at G, and bring back the Nos. 3 from G to H; then take the Nos. 4 at H, and place between the Nos. 4 at G, and bring back the Nos. 4 from G to H; then take Nos. 5 at E, and place between Nos. 5 at F, and bring back the Nos. 5 from F to E; then take the Nos. 6 at E, and place them inside of Nos. 6 at F, and bring back the Nos. 6 from F to E. Commence at A, as at first, and repeat until the braid is finished.

Braid this over a small wire, with a hole in one end like the eye of a needle, so as to draw a small cord in the place of the wire. When you have it braided, take off your weights, tie the ends fast on the wire, and push the braid together on the wire; then boil in water about ten minutes; then take it out, and put in an oven as hot as it will bear without burning, until it is quite dry; then take it out, and slip it off the wire on to the cord, and sew the ends of the braid so it will not slip on the cord, and put a little shellac on the end to keep it fast. If you want it elastic, use elastic cord. To vary the size of the braid, vary the number of hairs in a strand.

Twelve-Square Chain Braid.

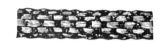

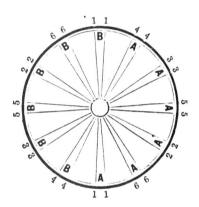

TAKE twenty-four strands, and place on table like pattern. Commence at A: take Nos. 1, and place between Nos. 1 at B, and bring back Nos. 1 from B and lay in place of Nos. 1 at A; then change the Nos. 2 at A and B the same way; then change the succeeding numbers, 3, 4, 5 and 6, all the same way. Then you are through the braid, ready to commence at Nos. 1 again, as at first, and repeat until the braid is the desired length.

Braid this over a small wire, with a hole in one end like the eye of a needle, so as to draw a small cord in the place of the wire. When you have it braided, take off your weights, tie the ends fast on the wire, and push the braid together; then boil in water about ten minutes; then take it out and put it in an oven as hot as it will bear without burning, until it is quite dry; then take it out and slip it off the wire on to the cord, sew the ends of the braid so it will not slip on the cord, and put a little shellac on the end to keep it fast. If you want it elastic, use elastic cord. To vary the size of the braid, vary the number of hairs in a strand.

Flat Twist Chain Braid.

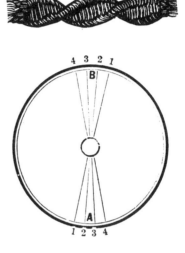

TAKE eight strands, with ninety hairs in a strand, and place them on table like pattern. Commence by taking No. 1 at A in right hand, and No. 1 at B in left hand, and swing around table to the right—the No. 1 in right hand over across Nos. 2, 3 and 4 at B, and the No. 1 in left hand over across Nos. 2, 3 and 4 at A. Repeat until the braid is finished.

Braid this over a small wire, with a hole in one end like the eye of a needle, so as to draw a small cord in the place of the wire. When you have it braided, take off your weights, tie the ends fast on the wire, and push the braid together; then boil in water about ten minutes; then take it out and put it in an oven as hot as it will bear without burning, until it is quite dry; then take it out and slip it off the wire on to the cord, sew the ends of the braid so it will not slip on the cord, and put a little shellac on the end to keep it fast. If you want it elastic, use elastic cord. To vary the size of the braid, vary the number of hairs in a strand.

Rib Chain Braid.

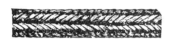

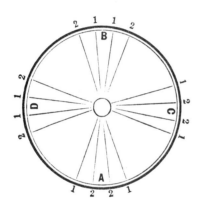

TAKE sixteen strands, eighty hairs in a strand, and place them on table like pattern. Commence at A: take both No. 1 strands, and cross over in between Nos. 1 on the opposite side to B; then bring back both Nos. 2 from B to A, and place them in between Nos. 2; then walk around table to C, and braid it across table to D, as before. Then commence at A, and repeat until braid is finished.

Braid this over a small wire, with a hole in one end like the eye of a needle, so as to draw a small cord in the place of the wire. When you have it braided, take off your weights, tie the ends fast on the wire, and push the braid together on the wire; then boil in water about ten minutes; then take it out, and put in an oven as hot as it will bear without burning, until it is quite dry; then take it out, and slip it off the wire on to the cord, and sew the ends of the braid so it will not slip on the cord, and put a little shellac on the end to keep it fast. If you want it elastic, use elastic cord. To vary the size of the braid, vary the number of hairs in a strand.

Fancy Cable Chain Braid.

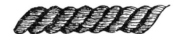

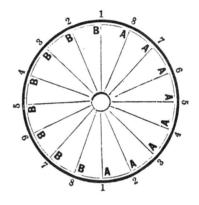

AKE any number of strands that can be divided by two, eight hairs in a strand, and place on table like pattern. Commence by taking Nos. 1 at A and B, and change places by swinging them to the right; then take Nos. 2 at A and B, and change places with them by swinging to the left; then take Nos. 3 at A and B, and change places by swinging them to the right; then Nos. 4, and change places by swinging them to the left, and so on, swinging to the right and left alternately, until the braid is finished.

Braid this over a small wire, with a hole in one end like the eye of a needle, so as to draw a small cord in the place of the wire. When you have it braided, take off your weights, tie the ends fast on the wire, and push the braid together; then boil in water about ten minutes; then take it out and put it in an oven as hot as it will bear without burning, until it is quite dry; then take it out and slip it off the wire on to the cord, sew the ends of the braid so it will not slip on the cord, and put a little shellac on the end to keep it fast. If you want it elastic, use elastic cord. To vary the size of the braid, vary the number of hairs in a strand.

Square Cable Chain Braid.

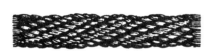

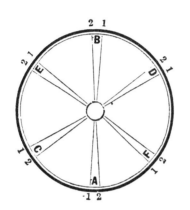

TAKE any number of strands that can be divided by two, with eighty hairs in a strand, and place them on table like pattern. Commence at A and B: take Nos. 1 and swing them around table to the right—No. 1 from A around to B across No. 2 at B, and No. 1 from B across No. 2 at A; then take Nos. 1 at C and D and change as before; then change the same at E and F and at B and A, and so on around the table to the right until the chain is completed. Any number of strands can be used by increasing the number in each place, or by having three, four, five or six in a place, care being taken to cross all the strands. For instance, there are four strands, No. 1 must be crossed over all as you braid around the table. By adding strands a different braid is formed.

Braid this over a small wire, with a hole in one end like the eye of a needle, so as to draw a small cord in the place of the wire. When you have it braided, take off your weights, tie the ends fast on the wire, and push the braid together; then boil in water about ten minutes; then take it out and put it in an oven as hot as it will bear without burning, until it is quite dry; then take it out and slip it off the wire on to the cord, sew the ends of the braid so it will not slip on the cord, and put a little shellac on the end to keep it fast. If you want it elastic, use elastic cord. To vary the size of the braid, vary the number of hairs in a strand.

Fob Chain Braid.

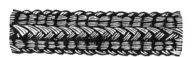

TAKE twenty strands, seventy hairs in a strand, and place them on table like pattern. Commence at A : cross No. 1 in the right hand over the No. 1 in the left hand, and then go to B and cross No. 1 in the left hand over No. 1 in the right hand ; then go back to A, and take Nos. 1 and cross inside of Nos. 1 at B, and bring back Nos. 1 from B to A ; then take Nos. 2, and

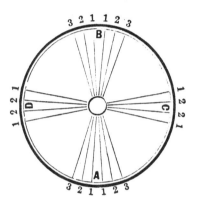

change the same ; then change Nos. 3 the same ; then go to C, and take Nos. 1 and cross inside of Nos. 2 at D, and bring back Nos. 1 from D and lay inside of Nos. 2 at C ; then commence at A, as at first, and repeat until the braid is finished.

Braid this over a small wire, with a hole in one end like the eye of a needle, so as to draw a small cord in the place of the wire. When you have it braided, take off your weights, tie the ends fast on the wire, and push the braid together on the wire ; then boil in water about ten minutes ; then take it out, and put in an oven as hot as it will bear without burning, until it is quite dry ; then take it out, and slip it off the wire on to the cord, and sew the ends of the braid so it will not slip on the cord, and put a little shellac on the end to keep it fast. If you want it elastic, use elastic cord. To vary the size of the braid, vary the number of hairs in a strand.

Square Ribbed Chain Braid.

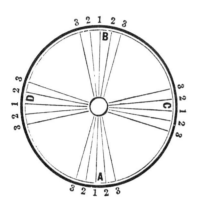

TAKE twenty strands, seventy hairs in a strand, and place them on table like pattern. Commence by taking No. 1 at A in right hand and No. 1 at B in left hand, swing to the right and change places with them; then take Nos. 3 at A, and lay inside of Nos. 2 at B, and bring Nos. 3 from B and lay inside of Nos. 2 at A; then go to C, and take No. 1 in right hand and No. 1 at D in left hand, swing to the right and change places with them; then take Nos. 3 at C, and lay inside of Nos. 2 at D, and bring back Nos. 3 from D and lay inside of Nos. 2 at C; then commence at A as at first, and repeat until the braid is finished.

Braid this over a small wire, with a hole in one end like the eye of a needle, so as to draw a small cord in the place of the wire. When you have it braided, take off your weights, tie the ends fast on the wire, and push the braid together; then boil in water about ten minutes; then take it out and put it in an oven as hot as it will bear without burning, until it is quite dry; then take it out and slip it off the wire on to the cord, sew the ends of the braid so it will not slip on the cord, and put a little shellac on the end to keep it fast. If you want it elastic, use elastic cord. To vary the size of the braid, vary the number of hairs in a strand.

Double Loop Chain Braid.

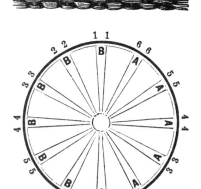

TAKE twenty-four strands, sixty hairs in a strand, and place them on table like pattern. Commence at A and B: take Nos. 1 at A, and lift them across the table, and lay the one in left hand between Nos. 1 at B, and the one in right hand on the outside of Nos. 1 at B, and bring back the Nos. 1 from B to A; then pass round the table to the right, and change (in the same manner), successively, the Nos. 3, 5, 6, 2, 4, 6, 2, 4, 5, 1, 3 and 5; then commence at A with Nos. 1, as at first, and repeat until the braid is finished.

Braid this over a small wire, with a hole in one end like the eye of a needle, so as to draw a small cord in the place of the wire. When you have it braided, take off your weights, tie the ends fast on the wire, and push the braid together; then boil in water about ten minutes; then take it out and put it in an oven as hot as it will bear without burning, until it is quite dry; then take it out and slip it off the wire on to the cord, sew the ends of the braid so it will not slip on the cord, and put a little shellac on the end to keep it fast. If you want it elastic, use elastic cord. To vary the size of the braid, vary the number of hairs in a strand.

Knot Chain Braid.

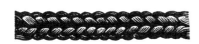

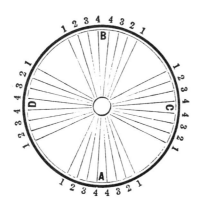

AKE thirty-two strands, fifty hairs in a strand, and place them on table like pattern. Commence at A: take Nos. 4, and lift over across table and lay outside of Nos. 1 at B; then bring back Nos. 4 from B and lay outside of Nos. 1 at A; then take Nos. 3 at A, and lift over across table and lay outside of Nos. 1 at B, and bring back Nos. 3 from B and lay outside of Nos. 1 at A; then change Nos. 2 at A and B the same; then take Nos. 1 and change the same; then go to D, and change the same as at A; then go to B, and change the same; then go to C, and change the same, and you are ready to commence again at A, as at first; repeat until braid is finished.

Braid this over a small wire, with a hole in one end like the eye of a needle, so as to draw a small cord in the place of the wire. When you have it braided, take off your weights, tie the ends fast on the wire, and push the braid together; then boil in water about ten minutes; then take it out and put it in an oven as hot as it will bear without burning, until it is quite dry; then take it out and slip it off the wire on to the cord, sew the ends of the braid so it will not slip on the cord, and put a little shellac on the end to keep it fast. If you want it elastic, use elastic cord. To vary the size of the braid, vary the number of hairs in a strand.

Double Rib Chain Braid.

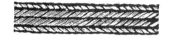

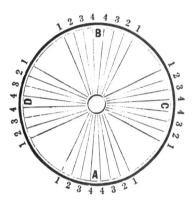

TAKE thirty-two strands, sixty hairs in a strand, and place them on table like pattern. Commence at A: take Nos. 4, and lift over table and lay outside of Nos. 1 at B, and bring back Nos. 4 from B and lay outside of Nos. 1 at A; then go to D, and change the Nos. 4 the same as at A and B; then go to B, and change the same as at A; then go to C, and change the same way; and then to A, and change as at first; and so on, repeating the changes until the braid is finished.

Braid this over a small wire, with a hole in one end like the eye of a needle, so as to draw a small cord in the place of the wire. When you have it braided, take off your weights, tie the ends fast on the wire, and push the braid together; then boil in water about ten minutes; then take it out and put it in an oven as hot as it will bear without burning, until it is quite dry; then take it out and slip it off the wire on to the cord, sew the ends of the braid so it will not slip on the cord, and put a little shellac on the end to keep it fast. If you want it elastic, use elastic cord. To vary the size of the braid, vary the number of hairs in a strand.

Fancy Chain Braid.

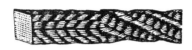

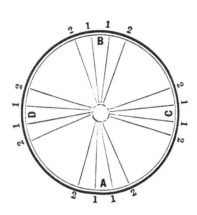

AKE sixteen strands, eighty hairs in a strand, and place them on table like pattern. Commence at A: change Nos. 1 across inside of Nos. 1 at B, and bring back Nos. 1 from B to A; then take Nos. 2 at A and change across inside of Nos. 2 at B, and bring back Nos. 2 from B to A; then go to C and change the Nos. 1 and Nos. 2 across with the numbers at D the same as at A; then return to A and commence as at first, and repeat ten times. Then change the figures on the table to correspond with the following diagram:

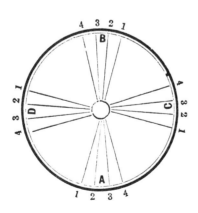

Then commence at A and B: take No. 1 at A in right hand and No. 1 at B in left hand, and swing around the table to the right, changing places with them; then take Nos. 1 at C and D and change the same; then change Nos. 2 at B and A the same; then change the Nos. 2 at D and C the same; then take the Nos. 3 at A and B and change the same; then change the Nos. 3 at C and D; then the Nos. 4 at B and A; then the Nos. 4 at D and C; then commence at A as at first, and repeat ten times; so on braiding alternately ten rounds, by the directions of each pattern, until the braid is finished.

Fancy Chain Braid.

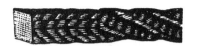

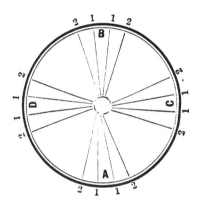

 AKE sixteen strands, eighty hairs in a strand, and place them on table like pattern. Commence at A: change Nos. 1 across inside of Nos. 1 at B, and bring back Nos. 1 from B to A; then take Nos. 2 at A and change across inside of Nos. 2 at B, and bring back Nos. 2 from B to A; then go to C and change the Nos. 1 and Nos. 2 across with the numbers at D the same as at A; then return to A and commence as at first, and repeat ten times. Then change the figures on the table to correspond with the following diagram:

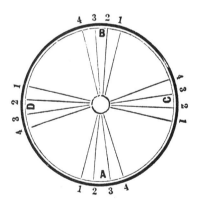

Then commence at A: take Nos. 1 and 2, lift across table to B and lay No. 1 outside of No. 4, and No. 2 between Nos. 1 and 2, and bring back Nos. 1 and 2 from B to A, and lay No. 1 outside of No. 4, and No. 2 outside of No. 1 at A; then go to C and take Nos. 1 and 2 and lift over table to D, and lay No. 1 outside of No. 4, and No. 2 between Nos. 1 and 2, and bring back Nos. 1 and 2 from C and lay No. 1 outside of No. 4 and No. 2 outside of No. 1 at C; then go to B and change the same; and so on around the table to the right, braiding alternately ten rounds, by each diagram, until the braid is finished.

Fancy Chain Braid.

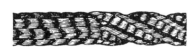

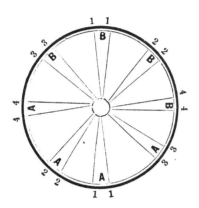

TAKE sixteen strands, eighty hairs in a strand, and place them on table like pattern. Commence at A: take Nos. 1, lift across the table and lay down inside of Nos. 1 at B, and bring back Nos. 1 from B to A; then lift Nos. 2 at A over inside of Nos. 2 at B, and bring Nos. 2 from B to A; then lift Nos. 3 from A to B, and bring back Nos. 3 from B to A; then lift Nos. 4 from A to B, and bring back Nos. 4 from B to A. Then change the figures on the table to correspond with the following diagram:

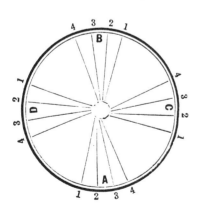

Then commence at A: take Nos. 1 and 2, lift across table to B, and lay No. 1 outside of No. 4, and No. 2 between Nos. 1 and 2, and bring back Nos. 1 and 2 from B to A, and lay No. 1 outside of No. 4, and No. 2 outside of No. 1 at A; then go to C and take Nos. 1 and 2 and lift over table to D, and lay No. 1 outside of No. 4, and No. 2 between Nos. 1 and 2, and bring back Nos. 1 and 2 from C, and lay No. 1 outside of No. 4 and No. 2 outside of No. 1 at C; then go to B and change the same; and so on around the table to the right, braiding alternately ten rounds, by each diagram, until the braid is finished.

Fancy Chain Braid.

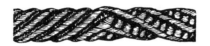

AKE sixteen strands, eighty hairs in a strand, and place them on table like pattern. Commence at A and B: take No. 1 at A in right hand and No. 1 at B in left hand, and swing around the table to the right, changing places with them; then take Nos. 1 at C and D and change the same; then change Nos. 2 at B and A the same; then change the Nos. 2 at D and C the same;

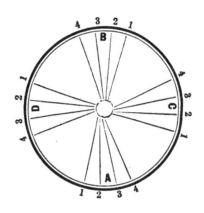

then take the Nos. 3 at A and B and change the same; then change the Nos. 3 at C and D; then the Nos. 4 at B and A; then the Nos. 4 at D and C—all the time swinging to the right. Braid around ten times.

Then commence at A: take Nos. 1 and 2, lift across table to B, and lay No. 1 outside of No. 4, and No. 2 between Nos. 1 and 2, and bring back Nos. 1 and 2 from B to A, and lay No. 1 outside of No. 4, and No. 2 outside of No. 1 at A; then change the same at C, B and D. Then commence again at A and braid ten rounds; so on braid-

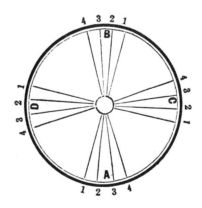

ing alternately ten rounds, by the directions of each pattern, until the braid is finished.

Fancy Chain Braid.

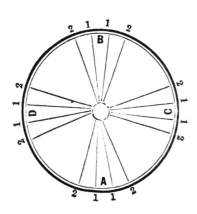

TAKE sixteen strands, eighty hairs in a strand, and place them on table like pattern. Commence at A: change Nos. 1 across inside of Nos. 1 at B, and bring back Nos. 1 from B to A; then take Nos. 2 at A and change across inside of Nos. 2 at B, and bring back Nos. 2 from B to A; then go to C and change the Nos. 1 and Nos. 2 across with the numbers at D the same as at A; then return to A and commence as at first, and repeat ten times. Then change the figures on the table to correspond with the following diagram:

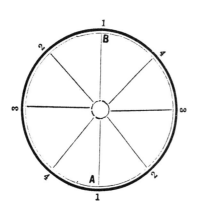

Take any number of strands that can be divided by two, eighty hairs in a strand, twenty strands for usual size, and place on table like pattern. Commencing, take No. 1 at A in right hand and No. 1 at B in left hand, and swing around the table to the right, and lay the one in right hand at No. 1 at B, and the one in left hand at No. 1 at A; then bring back No. 2 at B with right hand, and No. 2 at A with left hand, and swing around table to the left; then take No. 3 and swing to the right; then No. 4 and swing to the left; so on round, first to the right and then to the left, with every number of strands, till you get to No. 1. Braid ten rounds, alternately, by the directions of each pattern, until the braid is finished.

Fancy Chain Braid,

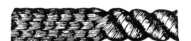

AKE sixteen strands, eighty hairs in a strand, and place them on table like pattern. Commence at A: take Nos. 1, lift across the table and lay down inside of Nos. 1 at B, and bring back Nos. 1 from B to A; then lift Nos. 2 at A over inside of Nos. 2 at B, and bring Nos. 2 from B to A; then lift Nos. 3 from A to B, and bring back Nos. 3 from B to A; then lift Nos. 4 from A

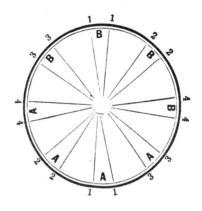

to B, and bring back Nos. 4 from B to A; then commence as at first and repeat ten times. Then change the figures on the table to correspond with the following diagram:

Take any number of strands that can be divided by two, eighty hairs in a strand, twenty strands for usual size, and place on table like pattern. Commencing, take No. 1 at A in right hand and No. 1 at B in left hand, and swing around the table to the right, and lay the one in right hand at No. 1 at B, and the one in left hand at No. 1 at A;

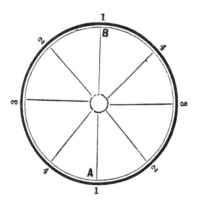

then bring back No. 2 at B with right hand, and No. 2 at A with left hand, and swing around table to the left; then take No. 3 and swing to the right; then No. 4 and swing to the left; so on round, first to the right and then to the left, with every number of strands, till you get to No. 1. Braid ten rounds, alternately, by the directions of each pattern, until the braid is finished.

Double Rib Chain Braid.

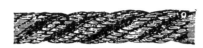

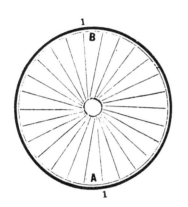

TAKE twenty-six strands, sixty hairs in a strand, and place them on table like pattern. Commence at A and B: Take Nos. 1 and change places by swinging them around the table to the left; then take the third strands to the right of A and B, and change places by swinging them around the table to the right; then take the fourth strands to the right of the ones last taken, and change places by swinging them around the table to the left, and so on, working around the table to the right; first swinging the strands to the left, and then to the right, taking alternately the third and fourth strands to the right of the ones last used, until the braid is finished.

Braid this over a small wire, with a hole in one end like the eye of a needle, so as to draw a small cord in the place of the wire. When you have it braided, take off your weights, tie the ends fast on the wire, and push the braid together; then boil in water about ten minutes; then take it out and put it in an oven as hot as it will bear without burning, until it is quite dry; then take it out and slip it off the wire on to the cord, sew the ends of the braid so it will not slip on the cord, and put a little shellac on the end to keep it fast. If you want it elastic, use elastic cord. To vary the size of the braid, vary the number of hairs in a strand.

Rope Chain Braid.

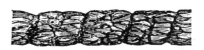

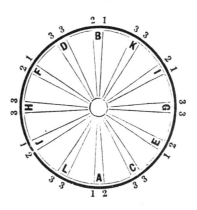

TAKE twenty-four strands, sixty hairs in a strand, and place them on table like pattern. Commence at A: take No. 2 in right hand, swing around the table to the right, and lay in place of No. 2 at B, and bring back No. 2 from B and lay in place of No. 2 at A; then take No. 1 at A in left hand, and change places with No. 1 at B, by swinging around to the left; then go to C, take Nos. 3, and lift over table and lay inside of Nos. 3 at D, and bring back Nos. 3 from D and lay in place of Nos. 3 at C; then go to E, and change the numbers at E and F the same as at A and B; then go to G, and change the same as at C and D, and so on, alternately changing, first as at A and B, and then as at C and D, until the braid is finished.

Braid this over a small wire, with a hole in one end like the eye of a needle, so as to draw a small cord in the place of the wire. When you have it braided, take off your weights, tie the ends fast on the wire, and push the braid together; then boil in water about ten minutes; then take it out and put it in an oven as hot as it will bear without burning, until it is quite dry; then take it out and slip it off the wire on to the cord, sew the ends of the braid so it will not slip on the cord, and put a little shellac on the end to keep it fast. If you want it elastic, use elastic cord. To vary the size of the braid, vary the number of hairs in a strand.

Diamond Shaped Chain Braid.

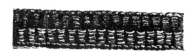

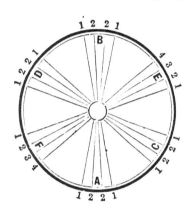

TAKE twenty-four strands, with seventy hairs in a strand, and place on table like pattern. Commence at A: take Nos. 2, lift across table and lay in between Nos. 2 at B, and bring back Nos. 2 from B to A; then take Nos. 1 at A, and lift across table and lay between Nos. 1 at B, and bring back Nos. 1 from B to A; then go to F, take No. 1 in right hand, swing around to the right and lay in place of No. 4 at E; then take No. 1 at E in left hand, and swing around to the left and lay in place of No. 4 at F; then go to C, take Nos. 2, lift across table and lay them in between Nos. 2 at D, and bring back Nos. 2 from D to C; then take Nos. 1 at C, lift across table and lay between Nos. 1 at D, and bring back Nos. 1 from D to C. Then you are through the braid, ready to commence as at first.

Braid this over a small wire, with a hole in one end like the eye of a needle, so as to draw a small cord in the place of the wire. When you have it braided, take off your weights, tie the ends fast on the wire, and push the braid together; then boil in water about ten minutes; then take it out and put it in an oven as hot as it will bear without burning, until it is quite dry; then take it out and slip it off the wire on to the cord, sew the ends of the braid so it will not slip on the cord, and put a little shellac on the end to keep it fast. If you want it elastic, use elastic cord. To vary the size of the braid, vary the number of hairs in a strand.

Fancy Square Chain Braid.

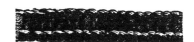

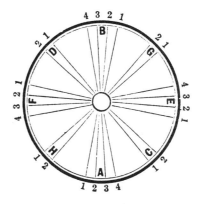

TAKE twenty-four strands, with eighty hairs in a strand, and place on table like pattern. Commence at A: take No. 1 in right hand, swing around to the right and lay in place of No. 4 at B; then take No. 1 at B in left hand, swing around table to the left and lay in place of No. 4 at A; then go to C, take No. 2 in right hand, swing around the table to the right and lay outside of No. 2 at D, and bring back No. 2 from D to C; then take No. 1 at C in left hand, swing around the table to the left and lay outside of No. 1 at D, and bring back No. 1 from D to C; then go to E, and change the numbers at E and F the same as you did at A and B; then change the numbers at G and H the same as you did at C and D. Then you are through the braid, ready to commence at A, as at first.

Braid this over a small wire, with a hole in one end like the eye of a needle, so as to draw a small cord in the place of the wire. When you have it braided, take off your weights, tie the ends fast on the wire, and push the braid close together; then boil in water about ten minutes, and take it out and put it in an oven as hot as it will bear without burning, until it is quite dry; then take it out and slip it off the wire on to the cord, sew the ends of the braid so it will not slip on the cord, and put a little shellac on the ends to keep it fast. If you want it elastic, use elastic cord. To vary the size of the braid, vary the number of hairs in a strand.

Fancy Square Chain Braid.

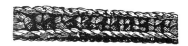

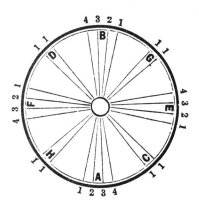

TAKE twenty-four strands, with eighty hairs in a strand, and place on table like pattern. Commence at A: take No. 1 in right hand, swing around to the right and lay in place of No. 4 at B; then take No. 1 at B in left hand, swing around table to the left and lay in place of No. 4 at A; then go to C, take Nos. 1 and lift them across the table and lay in between Nos. 1 at D, and bring back Nos. 1 from D to C; then go to E, and change the numbers at E and F the same as you did at A and B; then go to G, and change the numbers at G and H the same as you did at C and D. Then you are through the braid, ready to commence at A, as at first.

Braid this over a small wire, with a hole in one end like the eye of a needle, so as to draw a small cord in the place of the wire. When you have it braided, take off your weights, tie the ends fast on the wire, and push the braid close together; then boil in water about ten minutes, and take it out and put it in an oven as hot as it will bear without burning, until it is quite dry; then take it out and slip it off the wire on to the cord, sew the ends of the braid so it will not slip on the cord, and put a little shellac on the ends to keep it fast. If you want it elastic, use elastic cord. To vary the size of the braid, vary the number of hairs in a strand.

Fancy Square Chain Braid.

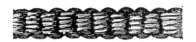

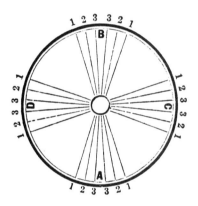

TAKE twenty-four strands, with eighty hairs in a strand, and place on table like pattern. Commence at A: take No. 1 at the left side of A in the right hand and No. 1 at the left of B in the left hand, swing them around the table to the right, and lay the one from B at the right of A and the one from A at the right of B; then go to C, take No. 1 at the left side of C in the right hand and No. 1 at the left of D in the left hand, swing them around the table to the right, and lay the one from C at the right of D and the one from D at the right of C; then go to B, take Nos. 3 and lift them across table and lay between Nos. 3 at A, and bring back Nos. 3 from A to B; then change Nos. 2 and 1 the same way; then go to C, take Nos. 3 and lift across the table and lay between Nos. 3 at D, and bring back Nos. 3 from D to C; then change Nos. 2 and 1 the same way. Then you are through the braid, ready to commence as at first, at A.

For explanation see page 9.

Fancy Square Chain Braid.

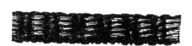

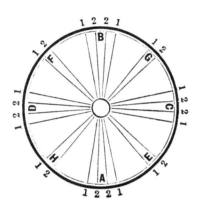

AKE twenty-four strands, with eighty hairs in a strand, and place on table like pattern. Commence at A: take Nos. 2, and lift across the table and lay between Nos. 2 at B, and bring back Nos. 2 from B to A; then change Nos. 1 the same way; then go to C, take Nos. 2 and lift them across the table and lay between Nos. 2 at D, and bring back Nos. 2 from D to A; then change Nos. 1 the same way; then go to E, take Nos. 1 and 2 and lift them across the table to F, and lay No. 1 from E at the right of No. 1 at F, and No. 2 from E at the right of No. 2 at F, and bring back the Nos. 1 and 2 from F to E; then go to G, and change the same from G to H, as you did at E and F. Then you are through the braid, ready to commence at A, as at first.

Braid this over a small wire, with a hole in one end like the eye of a needle, so as to draw a small cord in the place of the wire. When you have it braided, take off your weights, tie the ends fast on the wire, and push the braid close together; then boil in water about ten minutes, and take it out and put it in an oven as hot as it will bear without burning, until it is quite dry; then take it out and slip it off the wire on to the cord, sew the ends of the braid so it will not slip on the cord, and put a little shellac on the ends to keep it fast. If you want it elastic, use elastic cord. To vary the size of the braid, vary the number of hairs in a strand.

Fancy Twist Braid.

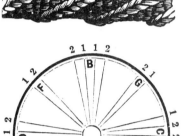

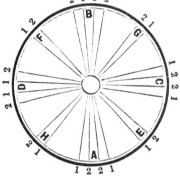

TAKE twenty-four strands, with seventy hairs in a strand, and place on table like pattern. Commence at A: take Nos. 1 across over and lay between Nos. 1 at B, and bring back Nos. 2 from B and lay between Nos. 2 at A; then go to E, take Nos. 1 and 2 and cross over to F, and lay No. 1 down at the right of No. 1 at F, and No. 2 at the right of No. 2 at F, and bring back Nos. 1 and 2 from F to E; then go to C, and change the numbers at C and D the same as you did at A and B; then go to G, and change the numbers at G and H the same as you did at E and F. Then you are through the braid, ready to commence at A, as at first.

Braid this over a small wire, with a hole in one end like the eye of a needle, so as to draw a small cord in the place of the wire. When you have it braided, take off your weights, tie the ends fast on the wire, and push the braid close together; then boil in water about ten minutes, and take it out and put it in an oven as hot as it will bear without burning, until it is quite dry; then take it out and slip it off the wire on to the cord, sew the ends of the braid so it will not slip on the cord, and put a little shellac on the ends to keep it fast. If you want it elastic, use elastic cord. To vary the size of the braid, vary the number of hairs in a strand.

Flat Chain Braid.

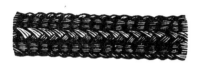

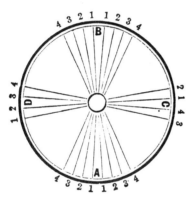

TAKE twenty-four strands, with seventy hairs in a strand, and place on table like pattern. Commence at A: take Nos. 1, and change places, by crossing one over the other; then go to B, and cross the Nos. 1 the same way; then go back to A, take Nos. 1 and cross over and lay between Nos. 1 at B, and bring back Nos. 1 from B to A; then take Nos. 2 at A, and cross over and lay between Nos. 2 at B, and bring back Nos. 2 from B to A; then change Nos. 3 and 4 the same way; then go to C, take Nos. 1 and 2 and cross over to D, and lay the No. 1 from C down at the left of No. 1 at D, and the No. 2 from C down at the left of No. 2 at D, and bring back the Nos. 1 and 2 from D to C; then take the Nos. 3 and 4, cross over to D, and lay the No. 3 from C down at the right of No. 3 at D, and the No. 4 from C down at the right of No. 4 at D, and bring back Nos. 3 and 4 from D to C.   Then you are through the braid, ready to commence at A, as at first.

For explanation, see page 9.

Necklace Pattern.

AKE sixteen strands, twenty hairs in a strand, and place them on table like pattern. Commence at A: take Nos. 1 and 4, lift across to B, lay in place of Nos. 1 and 4 at B, and bring back Nos. 1 and 4 from B to A; then take No. 2 at A in right hand and No. 3 in left hand, pass right hand round table to the right to B, and lay the No. 2 from A in place of No. 3 at B, and bring back

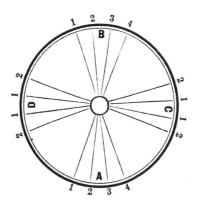

No. 2 from B to A in right hand, and pass left hand round table to the left, and lay No. 3 from A in place of No. 2 at B, and bring back No. 3 from B to A, and lay No. 3 from B down at No. 2 at A, and lay No. 2 from B down at No. 3 at A; then go to C, and take Nos. 1 across over inside of Nos. 1 at D, and bring back Nos. 1 from D to C; then go to A, and repeat this all three times; then the fourth time at C, you take Nos. 1 at C across over to D and lay outside of Nos. 2 at D, bring back the Nos. 1 from D to C and lay them outside of Nos. 2 at C. Then you are through the braid, ready to commence as at first at A. Braid it over a small cord, so as to put it up together.

Necklace Pattern.

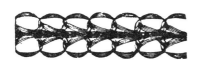

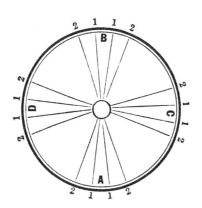

TAKE sixteen strands, twenty hairs in a strand, and place them on table like pattern. Commence at A: take Nos. 1 at A, lift across inside of Nos. 1 at B, and bring back Nos. 1 from B to A; then go to C, take Nos. 1 at C, lift across inside of Nos. 1 at D, and bring back Nos. 1 from D to C; then commence at A again, and repeat it three times; then commence at A, take Nos. 1 across to B and lay them outside of Nos. 2 at B, and bring back Nos. 1 from B to A and lay outside of Nos. 2 at A; then go to C, and change from C to D the same as from A to B; then you are through the braid, ready to commence as at first.

Braid this over a small wire, with a hole in one end like the eye of a needle, so as to draw a small cord in the place of the wire. When you have it braided, take off your weights, tie the ends fast on the wire, and push the braid together on the wire; then boil in water about ten minutes; then take it out, and put in an oven as hot as it will bear without burning, until it is quite dry; then take it out, and slip it off the wire on to the cord, and sew the ends of the braid so it will not slip on the cord, and put a little shellac on the end to keep it fast. If you want it elastic, use elastic cord. To vary the size of the braid, vary the number of hairs in a strand.

Necklace Pattern.

TAKE sixteen strands, twenty hairs in a strand, and place them on table like pattern. Commence at A: take Nos. 1 at A across over inside of Nos. 1 at B, and bring back Nos. 1 from B to A; then take Nos. 2 at A across over inside of Nos. 2 at B, and bring back Nos. 2 from B to A; then take No. 1 at C in right hand and No. 1 at D in left hand and change them, lay the No. 1 from

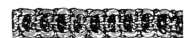

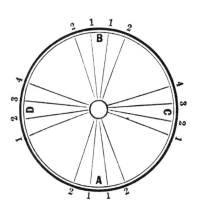

C in place of No. 1 at D, and lay the No. 1 from D in place of No. 1 at C; then change the Nos. 1 and 2 at A and B as at first; then change the Nos. 2 at C and D as you did the Nos. 1 at C and D; then change the Nos. 1 and 2 as before at A and B; then take Nos. 3 at C and D, and change as you did the Nos. 2 at C and D; then change again Nos. 1 and 2 at A and B as at first; then take the Nos. 4 at C and D, and change as you did the Nos. 3 at C and D. Then you are through the braid, ready to commence as at first.

Braid this without cord or wire.

Necklace Pattern.

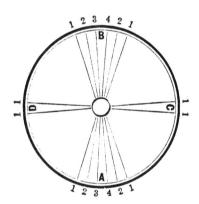

AKE sixteen strands, twenty hairs in a strand, and place them on table like pattern. Commence at A: take the Nos. 1, lift over to B, in place of Nos. 1 at B, and bring back Nos. 1 from B to A; then take Nos. 2 at A, and change over in place of Nos. 2 at B, and bring back Nos. 2 from B to A; then take No. 3 at A in right hand and No. 3 at B in left hand, and lay them inside of Nos. 1 at D, and bring back Nos. 1 from D and lay in place of Nos. 3 at A and B; then take No. 4 at A in left hand and No. 4 at B in right hand, and lay inside of Nos. 1 at C, and bring back Nos. 1 from C to A and B, and lay in place of Nos. 4; then commence as at first, and repeat this three times; then take Nos. 1 at A, lift over to B in place of Nos. 1 at B, and bring back Nos. 1 from B to A; then take Nos. 2 at A, and change over in place of Nos. 2 at B, and bring back Nos. 2 from B to A; then take Nos. 3 at A and B, lay inside of Nos. 1 at D; then take Nos. 4 at A and B, lay inside of Nos. 1 at C; then take Nos. 2 at A, and lay outside of Nos. 1 at B, and bring back Nos. 2 from B and lay outside of Nos. 1 at A; then take Nos. 1 at C, lift over inside of Nos. 1 at D, and bring back Nos. 1 from D and lay inside of Nos. 1 at C; then take No. 1 at C, on the side next to B, in right hand, and lay it inside of No. 1 at B; then take the No. 1 at D, next to B, in left hand, and lay it inside of No. 1 at B; then take the No. 1 at C, next to A, in right hand, and lay it inside of No. 1 at A; then take No. 1 at D, next to A, and lay it inside of No. 1 at A; then take the Nos. 3 and 4 at A, lift over to B, and lay outside of Nos. 1 at B, and bring back Nos. 3 and 4 from B and lay outside of Nos. 1 at A; then lift Nos. 2 at A over and lay in place of Nos. 2 at B, and bring back Nos. 2 from B to A, and lay in place of Nos. 2 at A; then take No. 4 at A in left hand and No. 4 at B in right hand, and lay them inside of Nos. 1 at C, and bring the Nos. 1 from C back in place of the Nos. 4 at A and B; then take No. 3 at B in left hand and No. 3 at A in right hand, and lay them inside of Nos. 1 at D, and bring back Nos. 1 from D and lay in place of Nos. 3 at A and B.   Then you are through the braid, ready to commence as at first.

Necklace Pattern.

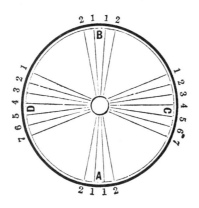

TAKE twenty-two strands, fifteen hairs in a strand, and place them on table like pattern. Have the strands at A and B black hair, and those at C and D light hair. Commence at A: take Nos. 1, and cross over inside of Nos. 1 at B, and bring back Nos. 1 from B and lay in place of Nos. 1 at A; then take Nos. 2 at A, cross over inside of Nos. 2 at B, and bring back Nos. 2 from B and lay inside of Nos. 2 at A; then take No. 1 at C in right hand and No. 1 at D in left hand, cross over and lay the No. 1 from C at D and the No. 1 from D at C; then change the Nos. 1 and 2 at A and B as at first; then take the Nos. 2 at C and D, and change them as you did the Nos. 1; then change again at A and B as at first; then take the Nos. 3 at C and D, and change as you did the Nos. 2; then change again at A and B, and so on till you get to Nos. 7, and after changing those, change again at A and B; then change Nos. 7 again, then those at A and B, then Nos. 6, then at A and B, then Nos. 5, and so on back to No. 1, and change No. 1 there as you did Nos. 7. Always braid those at A and B between each of those at C and D.

Necklace Pattern.

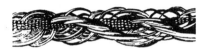

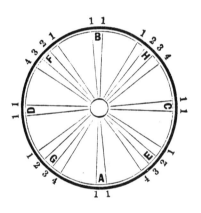

AKE twenty-four strands, with twenty-five hairs in a strand, and place on table like pattern. Commence at A: take Nos. 1, lift across inside of Nos. 1 at B, and bring back Nos. 1 from B to A; then go to C, and take Nos. 1 at C and cross inside of Nos. 1 at D, and bring back Nos. 1 from D to C; then go to A, and change Nos. 1 from A to B, as at first; then take Nos. 1 at E and F, and swing round table with the same, and lay down in between Nos. 1 at A and B, and lay the Nos. 1 at A and B in the place of Nos. 4 at E and F; then change the Nos. 1 at C across inside of Nos. 1 at D, and bring back Nos. 1 from D to C; then change Nos. 1 at A and B the same; then the Nos. 1 at C and D again; then take Nos. 1 at H and G, swing round table with the same, and lay in between Nos. 1 at C and D, and lay the right hand ones at C and D up in place of Nos. 4 at H and G; then you are through the braid, ready to commence as at first. Braid it over a cord, so as to push it together.

Necklace or Edging Braid.

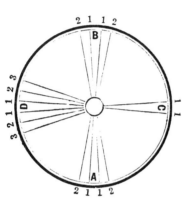

AKE sixteen strands, fifteen hairs in a strand, and place them on table like pattern. Commence at A: lift Nos. 2 across inside of Nos. 2 at B, and bring back Nos. 2 from B to A; then take Nos. 1 at A, lift across inside of Nos. 1 at B, and cross them, the one in right hand over the left, and bring back Nos. 1 from B to A, and cross the right over the left; then go to D, lift Nos. 1 across inside of Nos. 1 at C, cross the right over the left, and bring back Nos. 1 from C to D, and cross the right over the left; then repeat all from the beginning three times round the table; then go to D, lift Nos. 3, cross the right over the left, and lay them outside of Nos. 1 at C; then go to A, lift Nos. 2 across inside of Nos. 2 at B, and bring back Nos. 2 from B to A; then take Nos. 1 at A, lift across inside of Nos. 1 at B, cross the right over the left, and bring back Nos. 1 from B to A, and cross them; then go to D, lift Nos. 1 across inside of Nos. 1 at C, cross the right over the left, and bring back Nos. 1 from C to D; then take Nos. 3 at C, and lay inside of Nos. 2 at D, and leave them there. Then you are through the braid, ready to commence at A, as at first.

See explanation on page 9.

Head Dress or Necklace Braid.

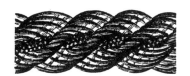

TAKE twenty-four strands, with eighty hairs in a strand, and place on table like pattern. Commence at A: lift Nos. 1 and 2 across inside of Nos. 1 and 2 at B, and bring back Nos. 1 and 2 from B to A; then go to C, lift Nos. 1 and 2 across inside of Nos. 1 and 2 at D, and bring back Nos. 1 and 2 from D to C; then go to A, and change the Nos. 1 and 2 from A to B, the same as at first; then take Nos. 1 at E and

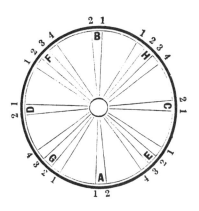

F, swing round table to the left, and lay them down between Nos. 1 and 2 at A and B; then lay the Nos. 2 at A and B in place of Nos. 4 at E and F; then change the Nos. 1 and 2 at C across inside of Nos. 1 and 2 at D, and bring back Nos. 1 and 2 from D to C; then change the same at A and B; then change again at C and D the same; then take Nos. 1 at H and G, swing round table to the left, and lay them between Nos. 1 and 2 at C and D, and lay the Nos. 2 at C and D in place of Nos. 4 at H and G. Then you are through the braid, ready to commence at A, as at first.

Braid it over a strong cord, and when braided push it close together, tie the ends, and boil in water five minutes; then heat it in an oven until it is quite dry, and it is ready for use.

Ring Pattern.

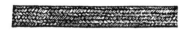

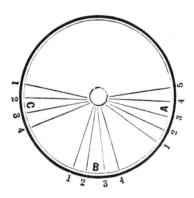

TAKE thirteen strands, fifteen hairs in a strand, and place them on table like pattern. Commence at A: lift No. 5 over between Nos. 2 and 3 at A; then take No. 1 at A and lift over between Nos. 2 and 3 at B; then take No. 1 at B and lift over between Nos. 2 and 3 at C; then lift No. 1 at C over between Nos. 2 and 3 at C; then lift No. 4 at C over between Nos. 2 and 3 at B, then lift No. 4 at B over between Nos. 2 and 3 at A. Then you are through the braid, ready to commence as at first, repeating until it is of the required length. Then tie it out straight on a flat stick, boil it in water five minutes; then heat it in an oven as hot as it will bear without burning, until it is quite dry, and then it is ready for use.

The above directions, after braiding, will suffice for finishing all Ring Braids, unless other directions are given.

Ring Braid.

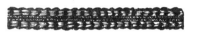

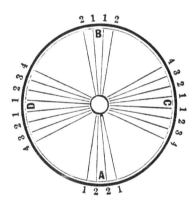

AKE twenty-four strands, with twenty hairs in a strand at C and D, and ten hairs in a strand at A and B, and place on table like pattern. Commence at A: take Nos. 1, and lift across table and lay inside of Nos. 1 at B, and bring back Nos. 2 from B and lay outside of Nos. 2 at A; then go to C, take Nos. 1, cross over and lay in between Nos. 1 at D, and bring back Nos. 1 from D to C; then take Nos. 3 at C, cross inside of Nos. 3 at D, and bring back Nos. 3 from D to C; then take Nos. 4 at C, cross over inside of Nos. 4 at D, and bring back Nos. 4 from D to C; then commence at A, and change them at A and B as at first; then go to C, and commence with the Nos. 2. You must leave the Nos. 1 every other time, and the Nos. 2 every other time, and braid it as at first.

Rib Ring Braid.

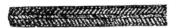

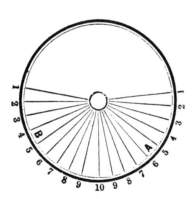

TAKE nineteen strands, twenty hairs in a strand, and place them on table like pattern. Commence at A: take No. 1, and lift over Nos. 2 and 3, under 4 and 5, over 6, 7, 8, 9 and 10, and lay over to B; then take No. 1 at B, lift over Nos. 2 and 3, under Nos. 4 and 5, over 6, 7, 8, 9 and 10, and lay over to A; then you are through the braid, ready to commence at A, as at first— first round to the left, and then to the right, and so on, repeating the changes as above, until the braid is finished. Then tie it out straight on a flat stick, boil in water five minutes, then heat it in an oven as hot as it will bear without burning until it is quite dry, and then it is ready for use.

Ring Pattern.

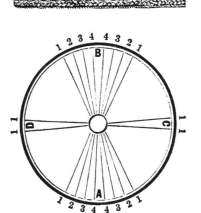

TAKE twenty strands, twenty hairs in a strand, and place them on table like pattern. Commence at A: take the Nos. 1, and lift across the table and lay in place of Nos. 1 at B, and bring back Nos. 1 from B to A; then take the Nos. 2, 3 and 4, and change the same; then go to C, take the Nos. 1 and lift across the table and lay in place of Nos. 1 at D, and bring back Nos. 1 from D to C; then commence again at A, take Nos. 1 and lift over the table and lay in the place of Nos. 1 at B, and bring back the Nos. 1 from B to A; then change the Nos. 2 and 3 the same as the Nos. 1; then go to C, and change the Nos. 1 over in the place of Nos. 1 at D, and bring back the Nos. 1 from D to C; then go to A, and take the Nos. 1, 2 and 3, and change the same as before; then go to C, and change the same as before. Then you are through the braid, ready to commence at A, as at first, and repeat until the braid is finished.

Ring Pattern.

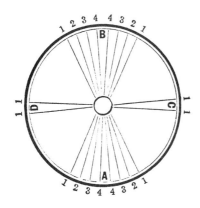

AKE twenty strands, twenty hairs in a strand, and place them on table like pattern. Commence at A: take Nos. 1, and lift over across the table and lay in place of Nos. 1 at B, and bring back Nos. 1 from B and lay in place of Nos. 1 at A; then take Nos. 2, 3 and 4, and change their places the same as Nos. 1; then go to C, take Nos. 1 and lift over across the table and lay in place of Nos. 1 at D, and bring back Nos. 1 from D to C; then go to A, take Nos. 1 and lift them over the table and lay in place of Nos. 1 at B, and bring back Nos. 1 from B to A; then take Nos. 3 and 4 and change the same; then go to C, take Nos. 1 and lift them over the table and lay in place of Nos. 1 at D, and bring back Nos. 1 from D to C. Then you are through the braid, ready to commence at A, as at first, and repeat the changes until the braid is finished.

Ring Pattern.

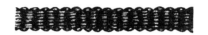

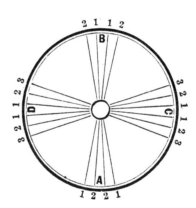

AKE twenty strands, fifteen hairs in a strand, and place them on table like pattern. Commence at A: take Nos. 1, lift across to B, and lay inside of Nos. 1, and bring back Nos. 2 from B and lay in between Nos. 2 at A; then go to G, take Nos. 1 and lift over inside of Nos. 1 at D, and bring back Nos. 1 from D to C; then take Nos. 2 at C, and cross over inside of Nos. 2 at D, and bring back Nos. 2 from D to C; then take Nos. 3 at C, cross over inside of Nos. 3 at D, and bring back Nos. 3 from D to C; then commence again at A, as at first, and repeat until it is braided the desired length.

When the braid is finished, tie it out straight on a flat stick, boil in water five minutes, and heat in an oven until perfectly dry, then it is ready for use.

Ring Pattern.

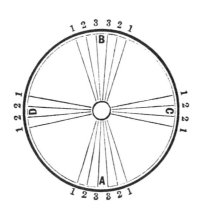

TAKE twenty strands, twenty hairs in a strand, and place them on table like pattern. Commence at A: take Nos. 1, and lift over table and lay in place of Nos. 1 at B, and bring back Nos. 1 from B to A; then take Nos. 2, and change the same; then the Nos. 3, and change the same; then go to C, take the Nos. 2 and lay outside of the Nos. 1; then go to D, and take the Nos. 2 and lay outside of the Nos. 1; then go to C, and take Nos. 2 and lift over table and lay in place of Nos. 2 at D, and bring back the Nos. 2 from D to C; then go to A, take Nos. 1 and lift across the table and lay in place of Nos. 1 at B, and bring back Nos. 1 from B to A; then take Nos. 3 at A, and lift across table in place of Nos. 3 at B, and bring back Nos. 3 from B to A; then go to C, take Nos. 2 and lay outside of Nos. 1; then go to D, take Nos. 2 and lay outside of Nos. 1; then go to C, take Nos. 2 and lift over table in place of Nos. 2 at D, and bring back Nos. 2 from D to C. Then you are ready to commence at A, as at first, and repeat until finished.

Ring Pattern.

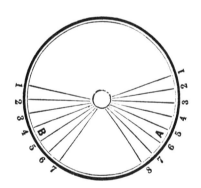

TAKE fifteen strands, twenty hairs in a strand, and place them on table like pattern. Commence at A: take No. 1, and lift over Nos. 2, 3 and 4, under Nos. 5, 6, 7 and 8, and pass it over to B; then take No. 1 at B, lift over Nos. 2, 3 and 4, under 5, 6, 7 and 8, and pass it over to A; then you are through, ready to commence at A, as at first, and repeat until the braid is finished— first round to the left, and then round to the right.

Ring Pattern.

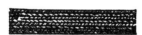

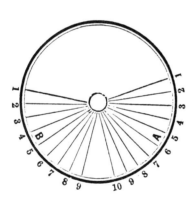

AKE nineteen strands, with ten hairs in a strand, and place them on table like pattern. Commence at A: take No. 1, and lift over Nos. 2, 3 and 4, under 5 and 6, over 7 and 8, under 9 and 10, and pass it over to B; then take No. 1 at B, and lift over Nos. 2, 3 and 4, under 5 and 6, over 7 and 8, under 9 and 10, and lay it over to A; then go to A and commence at No. 1, as at first, and repeat over and over, first to the left and then to the right, and so on until the braid is finished. Then tie it out straight on a flat stick, boil in water five minutes, and heat it in an oven as hot as it will bear without burning, until it is quite dry, and then it is ready for use.

Ring Pattern.

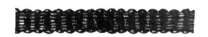

AKE twenty-four strands, and place on table like pattern. Commence at A: take Nos. 1 and lift across inside of Nos. 1 at B, and bring back Nos. 2 inside of Nos. 2 at A; then go to C, and take Nos. 1 and cross over inside of Nos. 1 at D, and bring back Nos. 1 from D to C; then take Nos. 2 at C, and cross over inside of Nos. 2 at D, and bring back Nos. 2 from D to C; then take Nos. 3

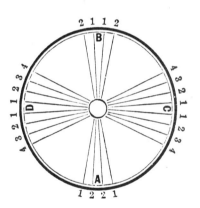

at C, and cross over inside of No. 3 at D, and bring back Nos. 3 from D to C; then take Nos. 4 at C, and cross over inside of Nos. 4 at D, and bring back Nos. 4 from D to C; if you wish to reverse every other time, you may leave the Nos. 1 and not braid them; then you are ready to commence at A as at first.

Ring Pattern.

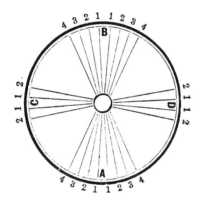

TAKE twenty-four strands, sixteen hairs in a strand, and place on table like pattern. Commence at A: take Nos. 1, and cross over to B, lay in between Nos. 1 at B, and bring back Nos. 1 from B and lay in place of Nos. 1 at A; then take Nos. 2 at A, and change them in the same way; then Nos. 3 the same; then Nos. 4 the same; then take Nos. 1 at C and D, and lift over Nos. 2; then lift Nos. 1 at C over in place of Nos. 1 at D, and bring back Nos. 1 from D to C; then go to A, and take Nos. 2, cross over between Nos. 2 at B, and bring back Nos. 2 from B to A; then take Nos. 3, and change the same way; then take Nos. 4, and change the same way; then go to C and D, and lift Nos. 1 over Nos. 2, and then lift over Nos. 1 at C and lay in place of Nos. 1 at D, and bring back Nos. 1 from D and lay in place of Nos. 1 at C; then you are ready to commence as at first at A, and repeat until the braid is finished. You will place double weight on the strands at C and D.

Ring Pattern.

TAKE twenty-eight strands, of twelve hairs in a strand, and place on table like pattern. Commence at A: take Nos. 1, and cross over the table and lay in place of Nos. 1 at B, and bring back Nos. 1 from B to A; then change the Nos. 2 the same; then take Nos. 4 at A, and lift over the table in place of Nos. 4 at B, and bring back Nos. 4 from B to A; then take Nos. 5, and change

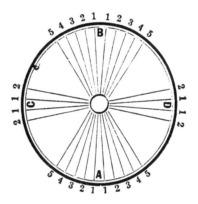

the same way; then go to C and D, and lift the Nos. 1 over the Nos. 2; then take Nos. 1 at C, and lift them over the table inside of Nos. 1 at D, and bring back the Nos. 1 from D and lay in place of Nos. 1 at C; then go to A, and take Nos. 1 and cross over in place of Nos. 1 at B, and bring back Nos. 1 from B to A; then take Nos. 2, 3, 4 and 5, and change all the same; then go to C and D, and lift Nos. 1 over Nos. 2; then lift Nos. 1 at C over the table, and lay them inside of Nos. 1 at D, and bring back Nos. 1 from D to C. Then you are through the braid, ready to commence at A, as at first, and repeat until the braid is finished. Place extra weight on the strands at C and D.

Ring or Bracelet Pattern.

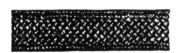

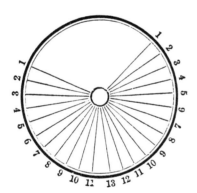

TAKE twenty-four strands, with twenty hairs in a strand, and place on table like pattern, thirteen on the right side and eleven on the left. Take No. 1 at right hand, lift over Nos. 2, 3 and 4, and under Nos. 5 and 6, and over No. 7; then take No. 1 again in right hand, and lift over Nos. 2, 3 and 4, and under Nos. 5 and 6; then take the same two that you have braided along, and lift over two strands, and under two, till you get to the center; then pass the same two strands across to the left side, and lay them down next to No. 11; then commence on the left side with No. 1, and braid the left side as you did the right; then the braid is through, ready to commence as at first, with No. 1 at right hand, and so on. Repeat till finished.

Ring Pattern.

TAKE thirteen strands, twelve hairs in a strand, and place them on table like pattern. Commence by lifting No. 7 over Nos. 6 and 5, and under Nos. 4 and 3, and over Nos. 2 and 1, and lay it next to No. 1 on the left side, making seven on the left side; then commence on the left side, take the outside one and braid it into the middle, over two and under two, till you get to the center, and lay it across on the opposite side. Then you are through the braid, ready to commence as at first, with the No. 7 at right hand. You can have any odd number of strands you please.

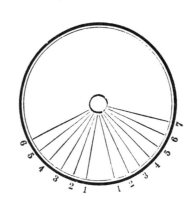

Ring Pattern.

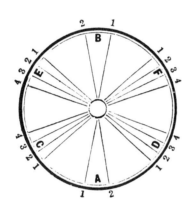

TAKE twenty strands, ten hairs in a strand, and place on table like pattern. Commence at A: take No. 2 in right hand, and swing it round the table to the right, and lay it across No. 2 at B, and bring back No. 2 from B to A; then take No. 1 at A in left hand, and swing it round the table to the left, and lay it across No. 1 at B, and bring back No. 1 from B to A; then commence at C and D: take No. 1 at C in left hand, and No. 1 at D in right hand, and change places with them by passing the left hand over the right; then take Nos. 2 at C and D, and change the same way; then take Nos. 3, and change the same way; then take Nos. 4, and change the same way; then go to B, and change the Nos. 1 at E and F as you did at C and D, by commencing at Nos. 1 first, then the Nos. 2, 3 and 4, in succession. Then you are through the braid, ready to commence as at first, at A. Braid it over a small wire.

Bracelet Tight Braid.

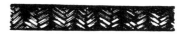

TAKE any number of strands that can be divided by four—sixty being the usual number—fifteen hairs in a strand, and place on table like pattern. Commence at A, with the inside row of figures: lift No. 3 over No. 2, and Nos. 1 and 3 over Nos. 2 and 4, and so on round table to the left till you get to A; then go to C, braid to the left, lift Nos. 1 and 2 over Nos. 3 and 4, and

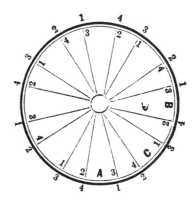

so on round to A; then commence at A, and braid round to the right, lift No. 2 over No. 3, and Nos. 3 and 4 over Nos. 2 and 1, and so on round table to A; then go to C, braid round to the right, and lift Nos. 2 and 4 over Nos. 3 and 1, and so on round to A. Then you are through the braid, ready to commence as at first.

Braid this over a round stick, the size you want the braid for use, varying the number of strands according to the size of the stick; then slip the braid from the stick on to the mold you wish to use, tying it so it will fit the mold exactly; and then boil in water five minutes, and take it out and put it in an oven as hot as it will bear without burning, until it is quite dry. Then it is ready for use.

Bracelet Braid.

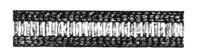

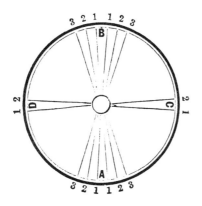

TAKE sixteen strands, thirty hairs in a strand, and place them on table like pattern. Commence at A: take the Nos. 1 and 2, and lay them over Nos. 3 right and left; then lay the Nos. 1 at A over Nos. 1 at C and D, and bring back the Nos. 1 from C and D and lay outside of Nos. 3 at A; then lay the Nos. 2 at A over Nos. 1; then go to B and repeat the same as at A, only change the Nos. 1 at B with the Nos. 2 at C, instead of the Nos. 1 at C; then lift the Nos. 1 at A over and lay between Nos. 1 at B, and bring back Nos. 1 from B to A; then go to C, and lift Nos. 1 and 2 over between Nos. 1 and 2 at D, and bring back the Nos. 1 and 2 from D to C.   Then you are through the braid, ready to commence at A, as at first.

Braid this over a small wire, and place double weight on the strands at C and D, and Nos. 1 at A and B.

Bracelet Braid.

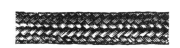

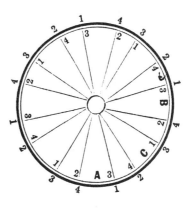

TAKE any number of strands that can be divided by four — forty being the usual number — twelve hairs in a strand, and place on table like pattern. Commence at A, with the inside row of figures: lift No. 3 over No. 2; then No. 1 over No. 2; then No. 4 over Nos. 3 and 2; then go to B, and change the same way, and so on round the table to A; then go to C, commence with the outside row of figures, and braid round to the left; lift No. 2 over No. 3; then No. 3 over No. 4; then No. 2 over No. 1; then No. 2 over No. 3, and so on round the table to A; then you will be through the braid, ready to commence as at first.

Braid this over a round stick, the size you want the braid for use, varying the number of strands according to the size of the stick; then slip the braid from the stick on to the mold you wish to use, tying it so it will fit the mold exactly; and then boil in water five minutes, and take it out and put it in an oven as hot as it will bear without burning, until it is quite dry. Then it is ready for use.

Elastic Bracelet Braid.

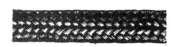

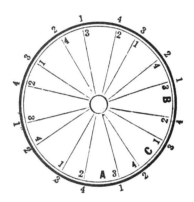

AKE any number of strands that can be divided by four—forty being the usual number for this braid—fifteen hairs in a strand, and place on table like pattern. Commence at A, with the inside row of figures: lift No. 2 in right hand, and put your left hand under the right hand and take Nos. 3 and 4, and bring them back and cross them over No. 1, and lay them all down; then go to B, and change the same way, and so on round the table to A; then go to C, commence with the outside row of figures, and braid round to the left; lift No. 3 in left hand, and put your right hand under the left hand and take Nos. 1 and 2, bring them back, cross them over No. 4, and lay them all down, and so on round the table to A. Then you will be through the braid, ready to commence as at first.

Braid this over a round stick, the size you want the braid for use, varying the number of strands according to the size of the stick; then slip the braid from the stick on to the mold you wish to use, tying it so it will fit the mold exactly; and then boil in water five minutes, and take it out and put it in an oven as hot as it will bear without burning, until it is quite dry. Then it is ready for use.

Elastic Bracelet Braid.

T AKE any number of strands that can be divided by four — sixty being the usual number for this braid—fifteen hairs in a strand, and place on table like pattern. Commence at A, with the inside row of figures, and braid round table to the right; lift No. 1 over No. 2, and No. 4 over Nos. 3 and 2; then repeat with the same strands, the No. 1 over No. 2, and No. 4 over Nos. 3 and 2; then go

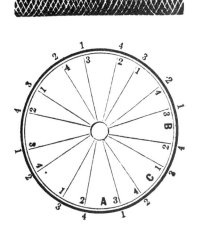

to B, and braid the same, and so on round table to A; then go to C, commence with the outside row of figures, and braid round table to the left; lift No. 1 over No. 2, and No. 4 over Nos. 3 and 2; then repeat, with the same strands, the same as you did at A and B, and so on round table to A. Then you are through the braid, ready to commence as at first. After it is braided, turn the braid inside out.

Braid this over a round stick, the size you want the braid for use, varying the number of strands according to the size of the stick; then slip the braid from the stick on to the mold you wish to use, and push it tight together, tying it so it will fit the mold exactly; and then boil in water five minutes, and take it out and put it in an oven as hot as it will bear without burning, until it is quite dry. Then it is ready for use.

Double Elastic Bracelet Braid.

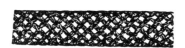

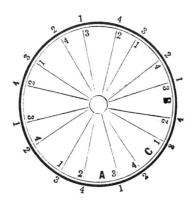

TAKE any number of strands that can be divided by four — sixty being the usual number for this braid — fifteen hairs in a strand, and place on table like pattern. Commence at A, with the inside row of figures, and braid round table to the right; cross No. 4 over No. 3, and No. 1 over Nos. 2 and 3; then repeat with the same strands; then go to B, and braid the same, and so on round table to the right, until you get to A; then go to C, and braid back round table to the left, by crossing No. 2 over No. 1, and No. 3 over No. 4, and No. 2 over No. 3; then repeat with the same strands, and so on round table till you get to A. Then you are through the braid, ready to commence as at first.

Braid this over a round stick, the size you want the braid for use, varying the number of strands according to the size of the stick; then slip the braid from the stick on to the mold you wish to use, and push it tight together, tying it so it will fit the mold exactly; and then boil in water five minutes, and take it out and put it in an oven as hot as it will bear without burning, until it is quite dry. Then it is ready for use.

Fancy Tight Bracelet Braid.

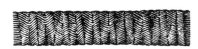

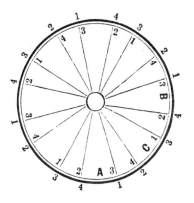

AKE any number of strands that can be divided by four—sixty being the usual number for this braid—fifteen hairs in a strand, and place on table like pattern. Commence at A, with the inside row of figures: lift No. 3 over No. 2, and Nos. 1 and 3 over Nos. 2 and 4; then go to B, and Braid the same to the left until you get to A; then commence at C, with the outside row of figures, and braid round table to the left again; lift Nos. 1 and 2 over Nos. 3 and 4, and so on round table till you get to A; then commence with the inside row of figures at A, and lift No. 2 over No. 3, and Nos. 2 and 4 over Nos. 3 and 1; then go to B, and braid the same to the right, and so on round table to A; then commence at C, with the outside row of figures, and braid round to the right; lift Nos. 3 and 4 over Nos. 2 and 1, and so on round table to A; then you are through the braid, ready to commence as at first. Be sure and braid the first two times round table to the left, and the last two to the right.

Braid this over a round stick, the size you want the braid for use, varying the number of strands according to the size of the stick; then slip the braid from the stick on to the mold you wish to use, tying it so it will fit the mold exactly; and then boil in water five minutes, and take it out and put it in an oven as hot as it will bear without burning, until it is quite dry. Then it is ready for use. To have it elastic, use elastic cord.

Reverse Tight Bracelet Braid.

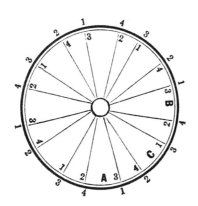

AKE any number of strands that can be divided by four — sixty being the usual number for this braid — fifteen hairs in a strand, and place on table like pattern. Commence at A, with the inside row of figures: lift No. 3 over No. 2, and No. 1 over No. 2, then No. 4 over Nos. 3 and 2; then go to B, and change the same to the left, and so on round table to A; then go to C, braid to the left with the outside row of figures, lift Nos. 3 and 4 over Nos. 1 and 2, and so on round to A; then commence again at A, and braid round to the right, lift No. 2 over No. 3, then No. 2 over No. 1, and Nos. 2 and 3 over No. 4, and so on round table to A; then commence at C, and braid to the right, lift Nos. 1 and 2 over Nos. 3 and 4, and so on round to A. Then you are through the braid, ready to commence as at first.

Braid this over a round stick, the size you want the braid for use, varying the number of strands according to the size of the stick; then slip the braid from the stick on to the mold you wish to use, tying it so it will fit the mold exactly; and then boil in water five minutes, and take it out and put it in an oven as hot as it will bear without burning, until it is quite dry. Then it is ready for use.

Banded Bracelet Braid.

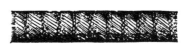

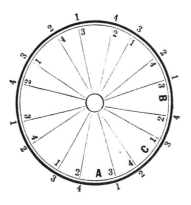

TAKE any number of strands that can be divided by four — sixty being the usual number for this braid — fifteen hairs in a strand, and place on table like pattern. Commence at A, with the inside row of figures: lift No. 3 over No. 2 and No. 1 over No. 2, then No. 3 over No. 4 and No. 3 over No. 2; braid round table to the left till you get to A; then repeat the same at C with the outside row of figures. After braiding the second time round, commence again at A, with the inside row of figures, and braid round to the right; lift Nos. 3 and 4 over Nos. 1 and 2, and so on round to A; then repeat at C with the outside row of figures. Then you are through the braid, ready to commence as at first.

Braid this over a round stick, the size you want the braid for use, varying the number of strands according to the size of the stick; then slip the braid from the stick on to the mold you wish to use, tying it so it will fit the mold exactly; and then boil in water five minutes, and take it out and put it in an oven as hot as it will bear without burning, until it is quite dry. Then it is ready for use.

Plain Open Braid.

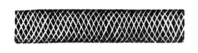

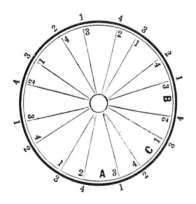

AKE any number of strands that can be divided by four—sixty being the usual number for this braid—fifteen hairs in a strand, and place on table like pattern. Commence at A, with the inside row of figures: lift No. 1 over No. 2, No. 4 over No. 3, No. 1 over No. 2, and No. 4 over No. 3; then No. 3 over No. 2, No. 1 over No. 2, and No. 4 over Nos. 2 and 3. Braid round table to the left till you get to A; then repeat the same at C; only braid the outside row of figures. Then you are through the braid, ready to commence as at first.

Braid this over a round stick, the size you want the braid for use, varying the number of strands according to the size of the stick; then slip the braid from the stick on to the mold you wish to use, tying it so it will fit the mold exactly; and then boil in water five minutes, and take it out and put it in an oven as hot as it will bear without burning, until it is quite dry. Then it is ready for use.

Open Fine Braid.

TAKE any number of strands that can be divided by four—eighty being the usual number for this braid—four hairs in a strand, and place them on table like pattern. Commence at A, with the inside row of figures: lift No. 2 over No. 3; then No. 2 over No. 1; then No. 2 over No. 3; then Nos. 2 and 3 over No. 4; then No. 2 over No. 1; then go to B, and change the same way,

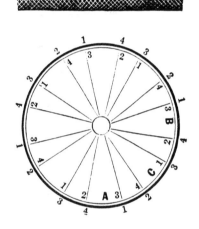

and so on round the table to A; then go to C, and commence with the outside row of figures, and change the same as you did at A, and so on round the table, when you will be through the braid, ready to commence at A, as at first.

Braid this over a round stick, the size you want the braid for use, varying the number of strands according to the size of the stick; then slip the braid from the stick on to the mold you wish to use, tying it so it will fit the mold exactly; and then boil in water five minutes, and take it out and put it in an oven as hot as it will bear without burning, until it is quite dry. Then it is ready for use.

Open Fine Braid.

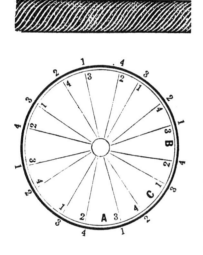

TAKE any number of strands that can be divided by four— eighty being the usual number for this braid—four hairs in a strand, and place them on table like pattern. Commence at A, with the inside row of figures: lift No. 1 over Nos. 2, 3 and 4; then No. 3 over Nos. 2 and 1; then No. 2 over Nos. 3 and 4; then No. 2 over No. 1; then go to B and change the same, and so on round the table to A; then go to C, and commence with the outside row of figures, and change the same as you did at A, and so on round the table, when you will be through the braid, ready to commence at A, as at first.

Braid this over a round stick, the size you want the braid for use, varying the number of strands according to the size of the stick; then slip the braid from the stick on to the mold you wish to use, tying it so it will fit the mold exactly; and then boil in water five minutes, and take it out and put it in an oven as hot as it will bear without burning, until it is quite dry. Then it is ready for use.

Open Lace Braid.

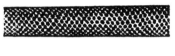

TAKE any number of strands that can be divided by four— sixty being the usual number for this braid—fifteen hairs in a strand, and place them on table like pattern. Commence at A, with the inside row of figures: lift No. 3 over No. 2, No. 3 over No. 4, No. 1 over No. 2, No. 3 over No. 2, and so on round the table to the left to A; then commence at C, lift No. 3 over No. 2, No. 3 over

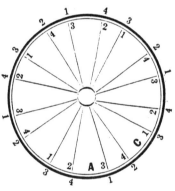

No. 4, No. 1 over No. 2, No. 3 over No. 2, No. 1 over No. 2, and No. 3 over No. 4. Then you are through the braid, ready to commence as at first.

Braid this over a round stick, the size you want the braid for use, varying the number of strands according to the size of the stick; then slip the braid from the stick on to the mold you wish to use, tying it so it will fit the mold exactly; and then boil in water five minutes, and take it out and put it in an oven as hot as it will bear without burning, until it is quite dry. Then it is ready for use.

Open Braid.

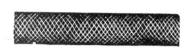

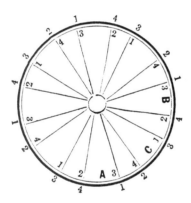

AKE any number of strands that can be divided by four— eighty being the usual number for this braid—four hairs in a strand, and place them on table like pattern. Commence at A, with the inside row of figures: lift No. 3 over No. 2, then No. 3 over No. 4, then No. 1 over No. 2, then No. 3 over No. 2, then No. 1 over No. 2, then No. 3 over No. 4; then go to B, and change the same way, and so on round the table to A; then go to C, and commence with the outside row of figures, and change the same as you did at A, and so on round the table, when you will be through the braid, ready to commence at A, as at first.

Braid this over a round stick, the size you want the braid for use, varying the number of strands according to the size of the stick; then slip the braid from the stick on to the mold you wish to use, tying it so it will fit the mold exactly; and then boil in water five minutes, and take it out and put it in an oven as hot as it will bear without burning, until it is quite dry. Then it is ready for use.

Basket Tight Braid.

TAKE thirty-two strands, or any number that can be divided by four, fifteen hairs in a strand, and place on table like pattern. Commence at A, with the inside row of figures, and braid round the table to the left; lift No. 3 over No. 2, No. 1 over No. 2, and No. 3 over No. 4; then commence at C, with the outside row of figures, and braid round the table to the left; lift Nos. 1 and 2 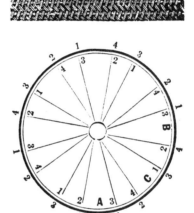 over Nos. 3 and 4; then commence at A, as before, and braid round the table to the right; put No. 3 under No. 2, and lift No. 2 over No. 1, and No. 3 over No. 4; then commence at C, as before, and braid round the table to the right, and put Nos. 1 and 2 under Nos. 3 and 4. Then you are through the braid, ready to commence at A, as at first.

Braid this over a round stick, the size you want the braid for use, varying the number of strands according to the size of the stick; then slip the braid from the stick on to the mold you wish to use, tying it so it will fit the mold exactly; and then boil in water five minutes, and take it out and put it in an oven as hot as it will bear without burning, until it is quite dry. Then it is ready for use.

Tight Braid.

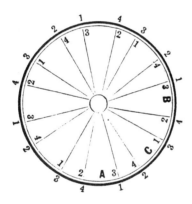

TAKE any number of strands that can be divided by four — forty being the usual number for this braid — twelve hairs in a strand, and place on table like pattern. Commence at A, with the inside row of figures, and lift Nos. 1 and 2 over Nos. 3 and 4; then go to B, and change the same way, and so on round table to A; then go to C, commence with the outside row of figures, and braid round to the left; lift Nos. 3 and 4 over Nos. 1 and 2, and so on round the table to A. Then you will be through the braid, ready to commence as at first.

Braid this over a round stick, the size you want the braid for use, varying the number of strands according to the size of the stick; then slip the braid from the stick on to the mold you wish to use, tying it so it will fit the mold exactly; and then boil in water five minutes, and take it out and put it in an oven as hot as it will bear without burning, until it is quite dry. Then it is ready for use.

Acorn Tight Braid.

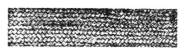

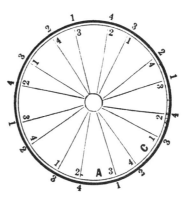

TAKE any number of strands that can be divided by four—sixty being the usual number for this braid—fifteen hairs in a strand, and place them on table like pattern. Commence at A, with the inside row of figures: lift No. 2 over No. 3, No. 4 over No. 3, No. 1 over No. 2, and No. 3 over No. 2, and so on round table to the right till you get to A; then commence at C, braid round to the right, lift Nos. 3 and 4 over Nos. 1 and 2, and so on round table to A. Then you are through the braid, ready to commence at A, as at first.

Braid this over a round stick, the size you want the braid for use, varying the number of strands according to the size of the stick; then slip the braid from the stick on to the mold you wish to use, tying it so it will fit the mold exactly; and then boil in water five minutes, and take it out and put it in an oven as hot as it will bear without burning, until it is quite dry. Then it is ready for use.

Half Tight Braid.

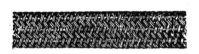

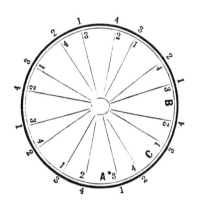

AKE any number of strands that can be divided by four — sixty being the usual number for this braid — fifteen hairs in a strand, and place them on table like pattern. Commence at A, with the inside row of figures: lift No. 3 over No. 2, and Nos. 1 and 3 over Nos. 2 and 4, and so on round table to A; then commence at C, with the outside row of figures, lift No. 2 over No. 3, No. 2 over No. 1, No. 2 over No. 3, Nos. 2 and 3 over No. 4, and No. 2 over No. 1, and so on round table to A. Then you are through the braid, ready to commence at A, as at first.

Braid this over a round stick, the size you want the braid for use, varying the number of strands according to the size of the stick; then slip the braid from the stick on to the mold you wish to use, tying it so it will fit the mold exactly; and then boil in water five minutes, and take it out and put it in an oven as hot as it will bear without burning, until it is quite dry. Then it is ready for use.

Fancy Tight Braid.

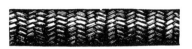

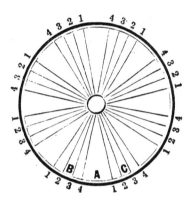

IN this pattern you braid with eight strands, or with two groups of fours. Commence at B: lift No. 4 in left hand, and lay down between Nos. 3 and 4 at C, and take No. 4 at C in right hand; then lift No. 3 at B over between Nos. 2 and 3 at C, and take No. 3 at C in right hand; then lift No. 2 at B over between Nos. 1 and 2 at C, and take No. 2 at C in right hand; then lift No. 1 at B over next to No. 1 at C, and take No. 1 at C in right hand, and then lift those in right hand over to B, and lay them all down; braid round to the right till you get to A; then take the next eight strands, and braid round table to the left; lift No. 1 at C over between Nos. 1 and 2 at B, and take No. 1 at B in left hand; then lift No. 2 at C over between Nos. 2 and 3 at B, and take No. 2 at B in left hand; then lift No. 3 at C over between Nos. 3 and 4 at B, and take No. 3 at B in left hand; then lift No. 4 at C over next to No. 4 at B, and take No. 4 at B in left hand, and then lift those in left hand over to C, and lay them all down; and so on round table, taking the next eight strands, till you get to A. Then you are through the braid, ready to commence as at first.

See explanation on page 100.

Plain Tight Braid.

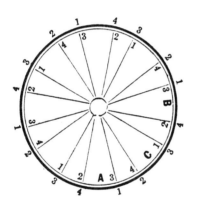

TAKE any number of strands that can be divided by four—eighty being the usual number for this braid—four hairs in a strand, and place them on table like pattern. Commence at A, with the inside row of figures: lift No. 3 over No. 2, then No. 3 over No. 4, then No. 1 over No. 2, then No. 3 over No. 2; then go to B, and change the same way, and so round the table to A; then go to C, and commence with the outside row of figures, and change the same as you did at A, and so on round the table, when you will be through the braid, ready to commence at A, as at first.

Braid this over a round stick, the size you want the braid for use, varying the number of strands according to the size of the stick; then slip the braid from the stick on to the mold you wish to use, tying it so it will fit the mold exactly; and then boil in water five minutes, and take it out and put it in an oven as hot as it will bear without burning, until it is quite dry. Then it is ready for use.

Acorn Braid.

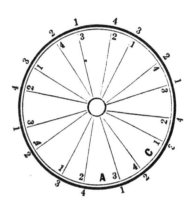

TAKE any number of strands that can be divided by four—sixty being the usual number for this braid—fifteen hairs in a strand, and place them on table like pattern. Commence at A, with the inside row of figures: lift No. 3 over No. 2, No. 3 over No. 4; No. 1 over No. 2, and No. 3 over No. 2, and so on round table to A; then go to C, take the outside row of figures, and make the same changes round to A, and repeat alternately at A and C, until the braid is long enough to cover the bottom of the acorn, and then commence at A, with the inside row of figures; lift No. 3 over No. 2, No. 3 over No. 4, No. 1 over No. 2, No. 3 over No. 2, No. 1 over No. 2, and No. 3 over No. 4, and so on round to A; then go to C, take the outside row of figures, and make the same changes round to A; then repeat until the braid is long enough to make the top or burr of the acorn. Then you are through the braid, ready to commence as at first.

Braid this over a round stick, the size you want the braid for use, varying the number of strands according to the size of the stick; then slip the braid from the stick on to the mold you wish to use, tying it so it will fit the mold exactly; and then boil in water five minutes, and take it out and put it in an oven as hot as it will bear without burning, until it is quite dry. Then it is ready for use.

Half Open Braid.

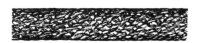

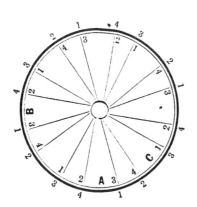

TAKE any number of strands that can be divided by four — sixty being the usual number for this braid—fifteen hairs in a strand, and place them on table like pattern. Commence at A, with the inside row of figures: lift No. 1 over between Nos. 2 and 3 at B; then lift No. 1 at B over between Nos. 2 and 3 of the next four strands, and so on round table to the left to A; then go to C, take the outside row of figures, lift No. 2 over No. 3, No. 2 over No. 1, Nos. 2 and 3 over No. 4; then No. 3 over No. 4, and No. 2 over No. 1, and so on round the table to the right, until the braid is finished.

Braid this over a round stick, the size you want the braid for use, varying the number of strands according to the size of the stick; then slip the braid from the stick on to the mold you wish to use, tying it so it will fit the mold exactly; and then boil in water five minutes, and take it out and put it in an oven as hot as it will bear without burning, until it is quite dry. Then it is ready for use.

Overshot Braid.

TAKE any number of strands that can be divided by four—sixty being the usual number for this braid—fifteen hairs in a strand, and place them on table like pattern. Commence at A, with the inside row of figures: braid to the right; lift No. 2 over Nos. 3 and 4, No. 1 over No. 2, and No. 3 over No. 2, and so on round to A; then go to C and repeat the same changes, with the outside row 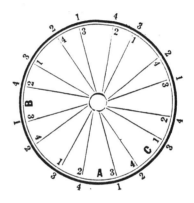 of figures, round to A; then commence at A with the inside row of figures, and braid to the left; lift No. 3 over Nos. 1 and 2, No. 4 over No. 3, and No. 2 over No. 3, and so on round to A; then go to C, and repeat the same changes, with the outside row of figures, round to A. Then you are through the braid, ready to commence as at first.

Braid this over a round stick, the size you want the braid for use, varying the number of strands according to the size of the stick; then slip the braid from the stick on to the mold you wish to use, tying it so it will fit the mold exactly; and then boil in water five minutes, and take it out and put it in an oven as hot as it will bear without burning, until it is quite dry. Then it is ready for use.

Diamond Tight Braid.

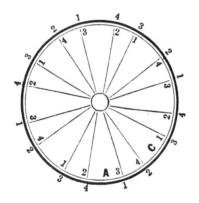

TAKE any number of strands that can be divided by four — sixty being the usual number for this braid — fifteen hairs in a strand, and place them on table like pattern. Commence at A, with the inside row of figures, and have Nos. 1 and 2 of white hair, and Nos. 3 and 4 of black hair: lift Nos. 1 and 2 over Nos. 3 and 4, and so on round table to the left, to A; then go to C, and braid round table to the right; lift Nos. 3 and 4 over Nos. 1 and 2, and so on round table to A. Then you are through the braid, ready to commence as at first.

Braid this over a round stick, the size you want the braid for use, varying the number of strands according to the size of the stick; then slip the braid from the stick on to the mold you wish to use, tying it so it will fit the mold exactly; and then boil in water five minutes, and take it out and put it in an oven as hot as it will bear without burning, until it is quite dry. Then it is ready for use.

Spiral Striped Braid.

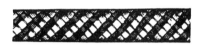

TAKE any number of strands that can be divided by four — sixty being the usual number for this braid — fifteen hairs in a strand, and place them on table like pattern. Commence at A, with the inside-row of figures, and have alternately four strands of white hair and four of black: braid round table to the left; lift Nos. 1 and 2 over Nos. 3 and 4, and so on round table to A; then go

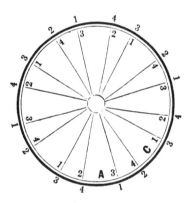

to C, braid round table to the right, lift Nos. 3 and 4 over Nos. 1 and 2, and so on round to A. Then you are through the braid, ready to commence as at first.

Braid this over a round stick, the size you want the braid for use, varying the number of strands according to the size of the stick; then slip the braid from the stick on to the mold you wish to use, tying it so it will fit the mold exactly; and then boil in water five minutes, and take it out and put it in an oven as hot as it will bear without burning, until it is quite dry. Then it is ready for use.

Empress Tight Braid.

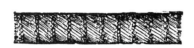

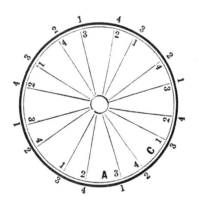

TAKE any number of strands that can be divided by four — sixty being the usual number for this braid — fifteen hairs in a strand, and place them on table like pattern. Commence at A, with the inside row of figures: lift No. 3 over No. 2, No. 1 over No. 2, No. 3 over No. 4, and No. 3 over No. 2; braid round table to the left till you get to A; then go to C, take the outside row of figures, and braid round to the right; lift Nos. 3 and 4 over Nos. 1 and 2, and so on round to A, and repeat with the inside row of figures, and then repeat again with the outside row. Then you are through the braid, ready to commence at A, as at first. Commence at C every other time, for you only braid the first change of figures once, and the last change three times.

Braid this over a round stick, the size you want the braid for use, varying the number of strands according to the size of the stick; then slip the braid from the stick on to the mold you wish to use, tying it so it will fit the mold exactly; and then boil in water five minutes, and take it out and put it in an oven as hot as it will bear without burning, until it is quite dry. Then it is ready for use.

Open Check Braid.

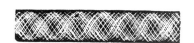

AKE any number of strands that can be divided by four — eighty being the usual number for this braid — four hairs in a strand, and place them on table like pattern. Have one-half the strands white and one-half black, and place on table alternately, four white and four black. Commence at **A**, with the inside row of figures: lift No. 2 over No. 3, No. 2 over No. 1, No. 2 over No. 3,

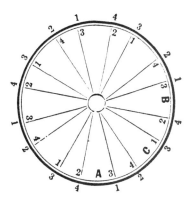

Nos. 2 and 3 over No. 4, and No. 2 over No. 1; then go to B, and change the same way, and so on round table to A; then go to C, commence with the outside row of figures, and change the same as you did at A, and so on round the table. Then you will be through the braid, ready to commence at A, as at first.

Braid this over a round stick, the size you want the braid for use, varying the number of strands according to the size of the stick; then slip the braid from the stick on to the mold you wish to use, tying it so it will fit the mold exactly; and then boil in water five minutes, and take it out and put it in an oven as hot as it will bear without burning, until it is quite dry. Then it is ready for use.

Scotch Plaid Braid.

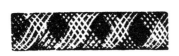

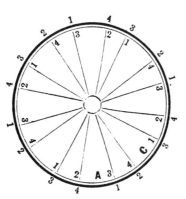

TAKE any number of strands that can be divided by four — eighty being the usual number for this braid — four hairs in a strand, and place them on table like pattern. Have one-third the strands white hair, one-third black, and one-third red, and place on table alternately, four white, four black, and four red. Commence at A, with the inside row of figures: lift No. 2 over No. 3, No. 2 over No. 1, No. 2 over No. 3, Nos. 2 and 3 over No. 4, and No. 2 over No. 1; then go to B, and change the same way, and so on round table to A; then go to C, commence with the outside row of figures, and change the same as you did at A, and so on round the table. Then you will be through the braid, ready to commence at A, as at first.

Braid this over a round stick, the size you want the braid for use, varying the number of strands according to the size of the stick; then slip the braid from the stick on to the mold you wish to use, tying it so it will fit the mold exactly; and then boil in water five minutes, and take it out and put it in an oven as hot as it will bear without burning, until it is quite dry. Then it is ready for use.

Half Open Braid.

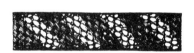

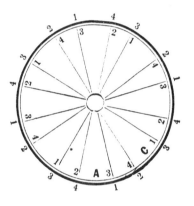

AKE any number of strands that can be divided by four — sixty being the usual number for this braid — fifteen hairs in a strand, and place them on table like pattern. Commence at A, with the inside row of figures: lift No. 3 over No. 2, No. 3 over No. 4, No. 1 over No. 2, and No. 3 over No. 2; braid half way round the table, and then braid the last half by lifting No. 3 over No. 2, No. 3 over No. 4, No. 1 over No. 2, No. 3 over No. 2, No. 1 over No. 2, and No. 3 over No. 4, and so on round to A; then go to C, and repeat the same. Then you are through the braid, ready to commence as at first.

Braid this over a round stick, the size you want the braid for use, varying the number of strands according to the size of the stick; then slip the braid from the stick on to the mold you wish to use, tying it so it will fit the mold exactly; and then boil in water five minutes, and take it out and put it in an oven as hot as it will bear without burning, until it is quite dry. Then it is ready for use.

Open Striped Braid.

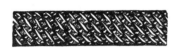

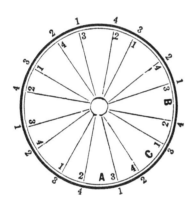

TAKE any number of strands that can be divided by four—eighty being the usual number for this braid—four hairs in a strand, and place them on table like pattern. Commence at A, with the inside row of figures, and have one-half the strands white hair and one-half black, and place alternately one strand of white and one strand of black: lift No. 2 over No. 3, No. 2 over No. 1, No. 2 over No. 3, Nos. 2 and 3 over No. 4, and No. 2 over No. 1; then go to B, and change the same way, and so on round table to A; then go to C, commence with the outside row of figures, and change the same as at A, and so on round table. Then you will be through the braid, ready to commence as at first.

Braid this over a round stick, the size you want the braid for use, varying the number of strands according to the size of the stick; then slip the braid from the stick on to the mold you wish to use, tying it so it will fit the mold exactly; and then boil in water five minutes, and take it out and put it in an oven as hot as it will bear without burning, until it is quite dry. Then it is ready for use.

Chinchilla Open Braid,

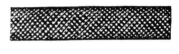

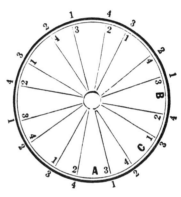

TAKE any number of strands that can be divided by four—eighty being the usual number for this braid—four hairs in a strand, and place them on table like pattern. Commence at A, with the inside row of figures, and have one-half of the strands white hair and one-half black, and place alternately two strands of white and two of black: lift No. 2 over No. 3, No. 2 over No. 1, No. 2 over No. 3, Nos. 2 and 3 over No. 4, and No. 2 over No. 1; then go to B, and change the same way, and so on round table to A; then go to C, commence with the outside row of figures, and change the same as you did at A, and so on round table; then you will be through the braid, ready to commence at A, as at first.

Braid this over a round stick, the size you want the braid for use, varying the number of strands according to the size of the stick; then slip the braid from the stick on to the mold you wish to use, tying it so it will fit the mold exactly; and then boil in water five minutes, and take it out and put it in an oven as hot as it will bear without burning, until it is quite dry. Then it is ready for use.

Fancy Lace Braid.

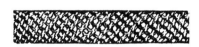

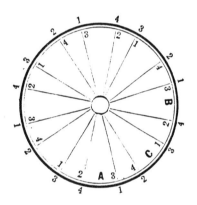

TAKE any number of strands that can be divided by four — eighty being the usual number for this braid — four hairs in a strand, and place them on table like pattern. Commence at A, with the inside row of figures, and have one-half of the strands white hair and one-half black, and place alternately two strands of white and two strands of black: lift No. 3 over No. 2, No. 3 over No. 4, No. 1 over No. 2, No. 3 over No. 2, No. 1 over No. 2, and No. 3 over No. 4; then go to B, and change the same way, and so on round to A; then go to C, commence with the outside row of figures, and change the same as you did at A, and so on round table. Then you will be through the braid, ready to commence at A, as at first.

Braid this over a round stick, the size you want the braid for use, varying the number of strands according to the size of the stick; then slip the braid from the stick on to the mold you wish to use, tying it so it will fit the mold exactly; and then boil in water five minutes, and take it out and put it in an oven as hot as it will bear without burning, until it is quite dry. Then it is ready for use.

Striped Elastic Braid.

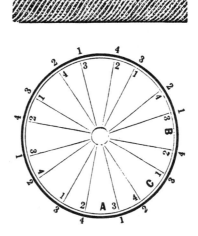

TAKE any number of strands that can be divided by four— sixty being the usual number for this braid—fifteen hairs in a strand, and place them on table like pattern. Commence at A, with the inside row of figures, and have one-half of the strands white hair and one-half black, and place alternately Nos. 1 and 2 of white and Nos. 3 and 4 of black: lift No. 1 over No. 2 and No. 4 over Nos. 3 and 2; then repeat with the same strands, the No. 1 over No. 2, and No. 4 over Nos. 3 and 2; then go to B and braid the same, and so on round table to A; then go to C, commence with the outside row of figures, and braid round to the left; lift No. 1 over No. 2, and No. 4 over Nos. 3 and 2; then repeat with the same strands, the same as at A and B, and so on round to A. Then you are through the braid, ready to commence as at first. After it is braided, turn the braid inside out.

Braid this over a round stick, the size you want the braid for use, varying the number of strands according to the size of the stick; then slip the braid from the stick on to the mold you wish to use, tying it so it will fit the mold exactly; and then boil in water five minutes, and take it out and put it in an oven as hot as it will bear without burning, until it is quite dry. Then it is ready for use.

Open Striped Braid.

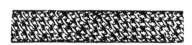

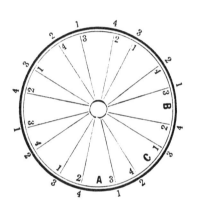

TAKE any number of strands that can be divided by four — sixty being the usual number for this braid — fifteen hairs in a strand, and place them on table like pattern. Commence at A, with the inside row of figures, and have one-half of the strands white hair and one-half black, and place alternately one strand of white and one of black; lift No. 1 over No. 2, and No. 4 over Nos. 3 and 2; then repeat with the same strands, the No. 1 over No. 2, and No. 4 over Nos. 3 and 2; then go to B, and braid the same, and so on round table to A; then go to C, commence with the outside row of figures, and braid round to the left; lift No. 1 over No. 2, and No. 4 over Nos. 3 and 2; then repeat with the same strands, the same as at A and B, and so on round to A. Then you are through the braid, ready to commence as at first. After it is braided, turn the braid inside out.

Braid this over a round stick the size you want the braid for use, varying the number of strands according to the size of the stick; then slip the braid from the stick on to the mold you wish to use, tying it so it will fit the mold exactly; and then boil in water five minutes, and take it out and put it in an oven as hot as it will bear without burning, until it is quite dry. Then it is ready for use.

Wide Striped Braid.

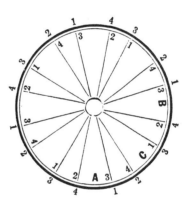

TAKE any number of strands that can be divided by four— eighty being the usual number for this braid—four hairs in a strand, and place them on table like pattern. Commence at A, with the inside row of figures, and have one-fourth of the strands white hair and three-fourths black, and place all the white strands on one side of the table and all of the black on the other side: lift No. 2 over No. 3, No. 2 over No. 1, No. 2 over No. 3, Nos. 2 and 3 over No. 4, and No. 2 over No. 1; then go to B, and change the same way, and so on round table to A; then go to C, commence with the outside row of figures, and change the same as at A, and so on round table. Then you are through the braid, ready to commence as at first.

Braid this over a round stick, the size you want the braid for use, varying the number of strands according to the size of the stick; then slip the braid from the stick on to the mold you wish to use, tying it so it will fit the mold exactly; and then boil in water five minutes, and take it out and put it in an oven as hot as it will bear without burning, until it is quite dry. Then it is ready for use.

Neapolitan Tight Braid.

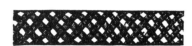

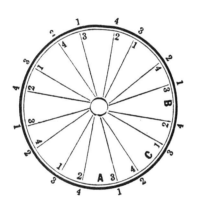

TAKE any number of strands that can be divided by four—eighty being the usual number for this braid—four hairs in a strand, and place them on table like pattern. Commence at A, with the inside row of figures, and have one-fourth of the strands white hair and three-fourths black—the Nos. 1 white and the Nos. 2, 3 and 4 black; lift No. 3 over No. 2, No. 3 over No. 4, No. 1 over No. 2, and No. 3 over No. 2; then go to B and change the same way, and so on round table to A; then go to C, commence with the outside row of figures, and change the same as at A, and so on round table. Then you are through the braid, ready to commence as at first.

Braid this over a round stick, the size you want the braid for use, varying the number of strands according to the size of the stick; then slip the braid from the stick on to the mold you wish to use, tying it so it will fit the mold exactly; and then boil in water five minutes, and take it out and put it in an oven as hot as it will bear without burning, until it is quite dry. Then it is ready for use.

Open Braid.

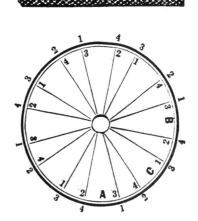

AKE any number of strands that can be divided by four—eighty being the usual number for this braid—four hairs in a strand, and place them on table like pattern. Commence at A, with the inside row of figures: lift No. 3 over No. 2, then No. 3 over No. 4, then No. 1 over No. 2, then No. 3 over No. 2; then go to B, and change the same way, and so on round the table to A; then go to C, and commence with the outside row of figures, and change the same as you did at A, and so on round the table, when you will be through the braid, ready to commence at A, as at first.

Braid this over a round stick, the size you want the braid for use, varying the number of strands according to the size of the stick; then slip the braid from the stick on to the mold you wish to use, tying it so it will fit the mold exactly; and then boil in water five minutes, and take it out and put it in an oven as hot as it will bear without burning, until it is quite dry. Then it is ready for use.

Explanations on Bracelets.

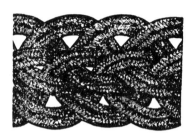

No. 1.

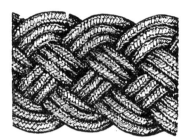

No. 2.

The above cuts represent the completed Bracelet Braid.   The No. 1 is formed from fourteen small braids, braided according to diagram and explanation on page 120 —using, however, but thirty-two strands, instead of eighty.

After you have the small braids all completed and prepared, as required in the explanation, sew them together at one end, so they all lie smooth and flat; then divide them off in twos, using each two as one strand, and plait then together; commence at the right side, take one strand at a time, and lift over one and under two until you get to the center, then commence on the left side and braid the same way, and so on till finished.   Then sew the ends well, trim them, and put on a little shellac to fasten them in the clasps.

No. 2 is from the same pattern, and is prepared and finished up in the same manner.   For this bracelet you use fifteen small braids; divide them into threes for each strand, and lift over one and under one. from each side to the center.

Explanations on Bracelets.

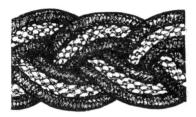 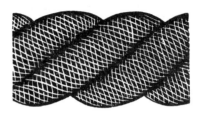

No. 1.   No. 2.

The No 1 cut of the above Bracelet Braids is formed from patterns on pages 103 and 113, and instead of using forty and sixty strands, use but thirty-two for each. Braid six small braids from pattern on page 103, and three from pattern on page 113. Sew them tight together at one end, divide them off in threes, with the open work braid between the two tight ones, use each three as one strand, and plait them together in a common three strand braid.

No. 2 is braided according to pattern on page 105. Have three of the braids; sew them fast at one end, and then twist them carefully and evenly together; then sew and fasten with shellac, and it is ready to be gold mounted.

Explanations on Bracelets.

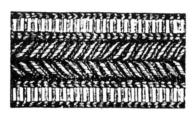

No. 1.

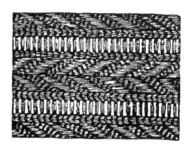

No. 2.

The No. 1 cut of the above Bracelet Braids, is formed from patterns on pages 42 and 102. Have two small braids from each of the patterns, lay them side by side, as in cut, and sew them firmly together, either with some of the hair, or with very fine silk of the same color. Then sew and trim the ends, and fasten with shellac.

No. 2 is braided from patterns on pages 34 and 102. Have four small braids like pattern on page 34, and two like pattern on page 102. Place them side by side, as in cut, and prepare and finish up the same as in the above.

Explanations on Bracelets.

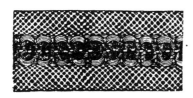

No. 1.

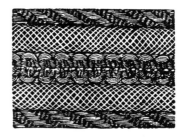

No. 2.

The patterns used for the No. 1, represented above, are found on pages 79 and 111. Have one braid from pattern on page 79, and two from that on page 111. Place them side by side, as in cut, and sew the ends firmly together, either with some of the hair, or with very fine silk of the same color. Then sew and trim the ends, and fasten with shellac.

For the No. 2, use two small braids from pattern on page 34, one from pattern on page 79, and two from pattern on page 111. Place them as in cut, sew them together, and prepare the same as No. 1.

Explanations on Bracelets.

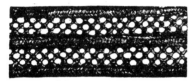 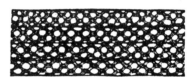

No. 1.   No. 2.

The No. 1 of the above Bracelet Braids is made up of two small braids from pattern on page 113, and three from pattern on page 117, using, however, but thirty-two strands, instead of sixty. Place them side by side, as in cut, and sew them together with some of the hair, or with fine silk of the same color. Sew, trim and shellac the ends, and they are ready to be gold mounted.

No. 2 is formed of four small braids, from pattern on page 113, and is prepared, sewed and finished up the same as No 1.

Designs in Hair-Work.

THE following designs of Hair Jewelry, Flowers and Pictures, are given for the purpose of showing a few of the many beautiful forms into which the human hair may be transposed. Each and every one of the devices on the following pages, with the exception of the flowers and pictures, can be braided from the diagrams and explanations given in the first one hundred and twenty pages of this book. Select any article you may wish to make, and by referring to the patterns, you can easily find the style and directions whereby to braid it. We might have given twice the number of patterns, or even more, but any person can, after a little experience, readily invent new and different styles of braids, and by so doing can satisfy their own peculiar tastes.

The making of Hair Flowers is very simple, and yet, of course, every one has first to learn it. Supply yourself with as many different colors of hair as you can, and by applying gum tragacanth it renders it capable of being cut in any shape you may wish—such as leaves, twigs, buds, etc, and by judiciously arranging the colors, the effect will be very pleasing. Pictures are made in the same manner, and any one possessing the least artistic skill can make any flower or picture desired, and many pleasing adornments and lasting mementos may thereby be had.

All articles intended to be worn as jewelry, should, of course, be mounted with gold, and as this kind of work is not done in all jewelry establishments, I wish to say that my facilities for this branch of business is complete, and the work is done in the best possible manner. I can guarantee satisfaction in all cases, let the style desired be what it may. In sending braids to be mounted, draw on paper, as near as can be, the style or design you want.

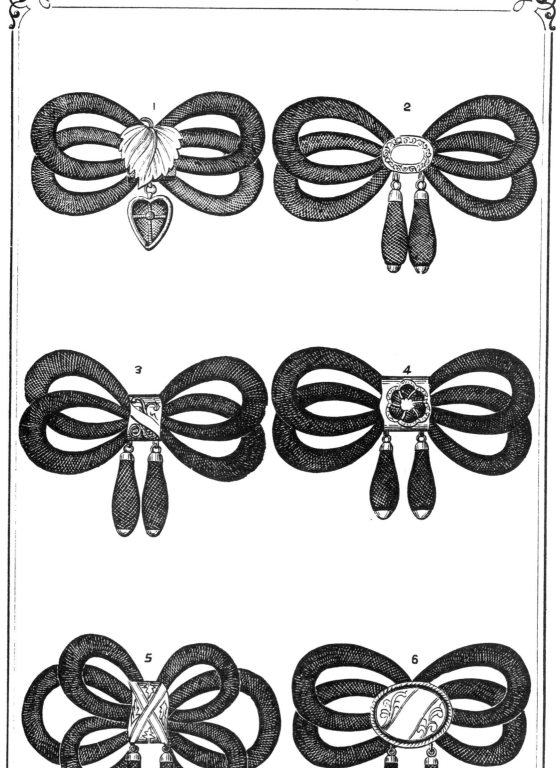

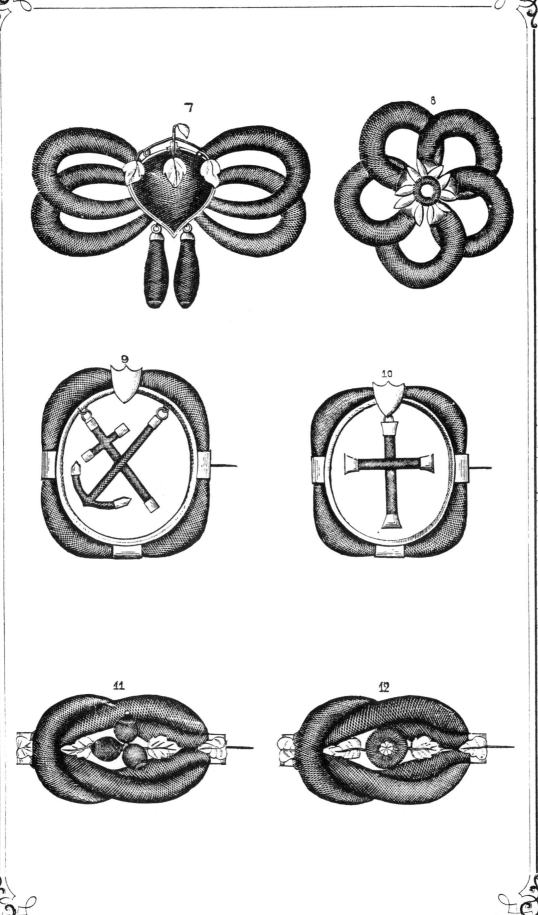

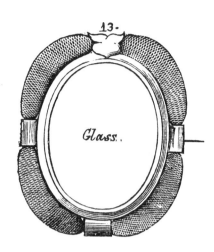

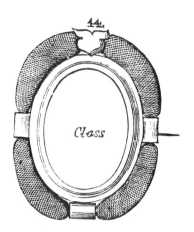

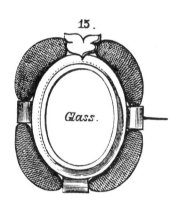

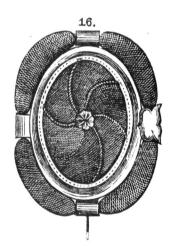

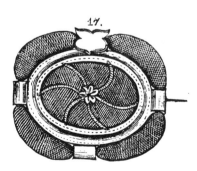

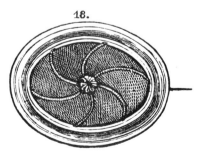

19

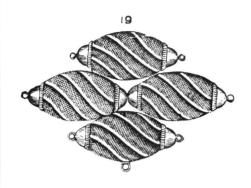

20

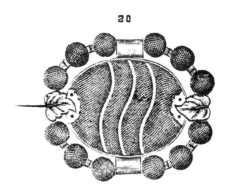

21

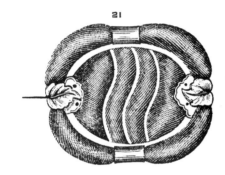

22

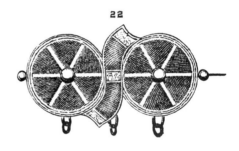

23

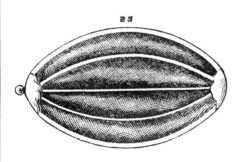

24

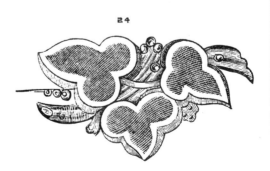

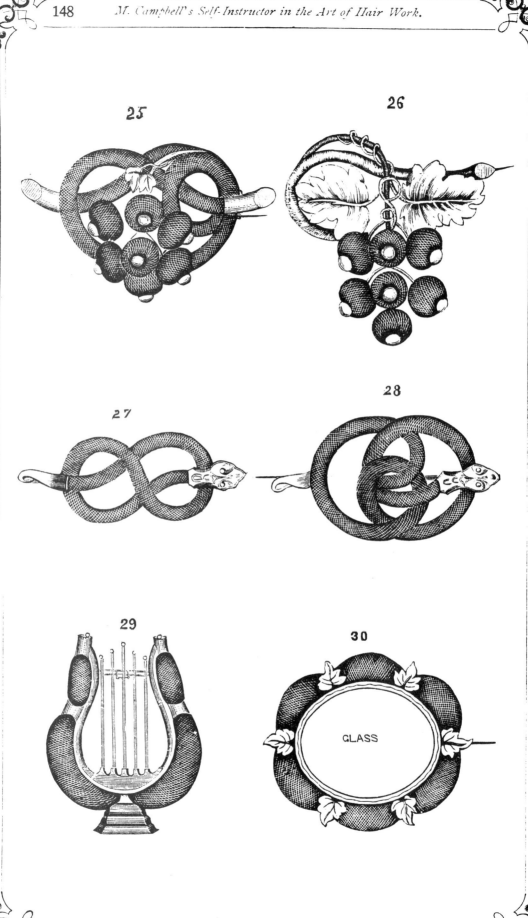

25

26

27

28

29

30

31

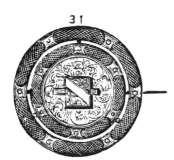

32

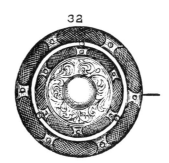

33

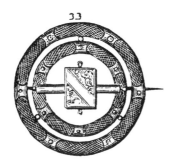

34

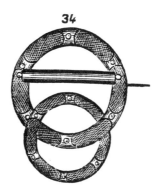

35

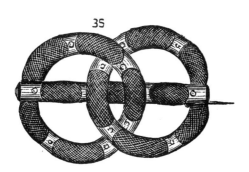

36

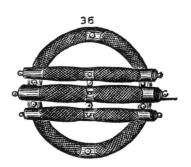

37.

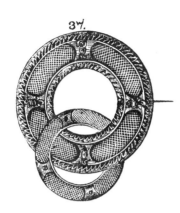

38

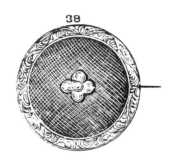

39.

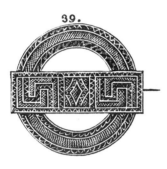

40.

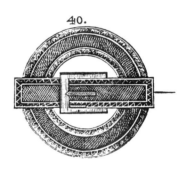

41.

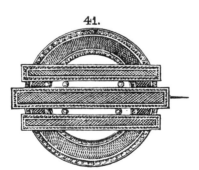

42.

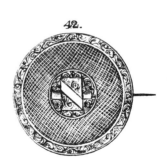

43

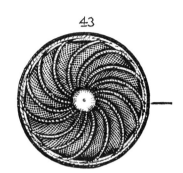

44

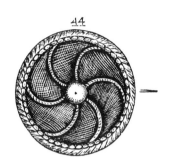

45

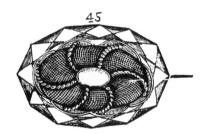

46

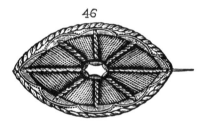

47

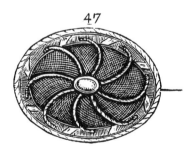

48

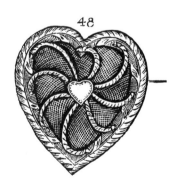

49

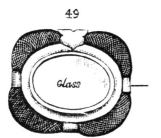

50

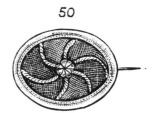

51

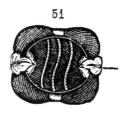

52

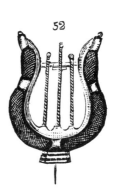

53

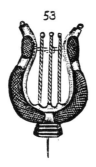

54

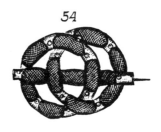

55

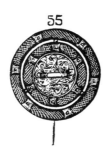

56

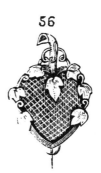

57

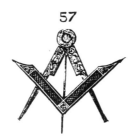

58

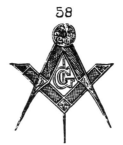

59

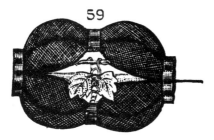

60

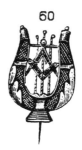

61

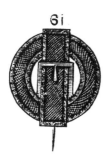

62

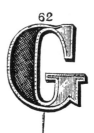

63

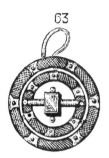

64

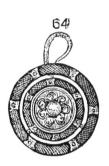

65

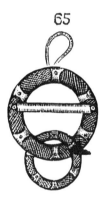

66

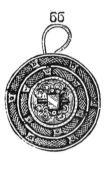

67

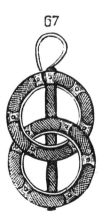

68

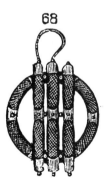

69

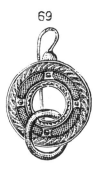

70

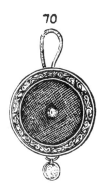

71

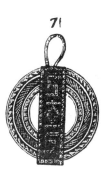

72

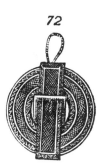

73

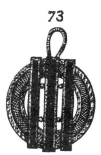

71

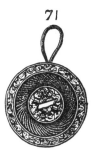

75

76

77

78

79

80

81

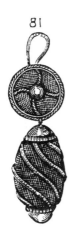

82

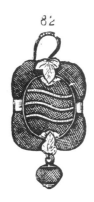

83

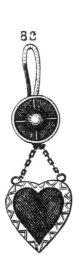

84

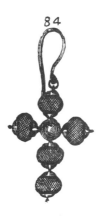

85

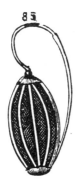

86

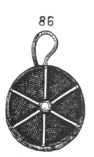

87

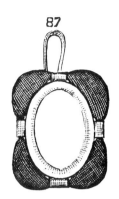

88

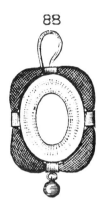

89

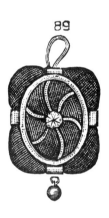

90

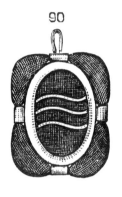

91

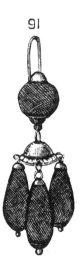

92

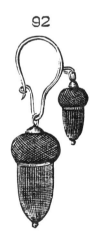

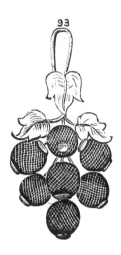

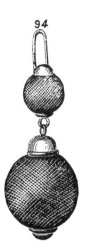

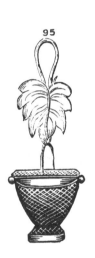

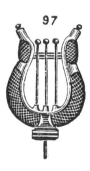

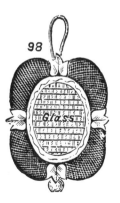

99

100

101

102

104

103

105
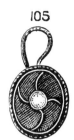

106
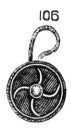

107
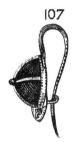

108
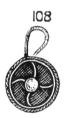

109
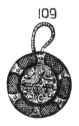

110
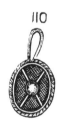

111
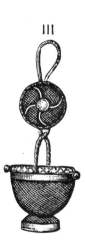

112
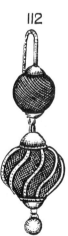

116

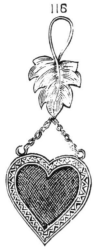

114

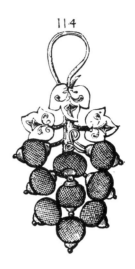

115

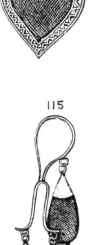

116

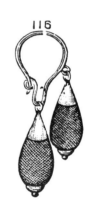

117

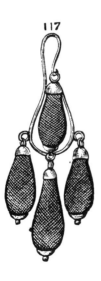

118

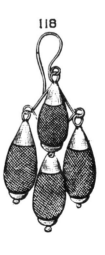

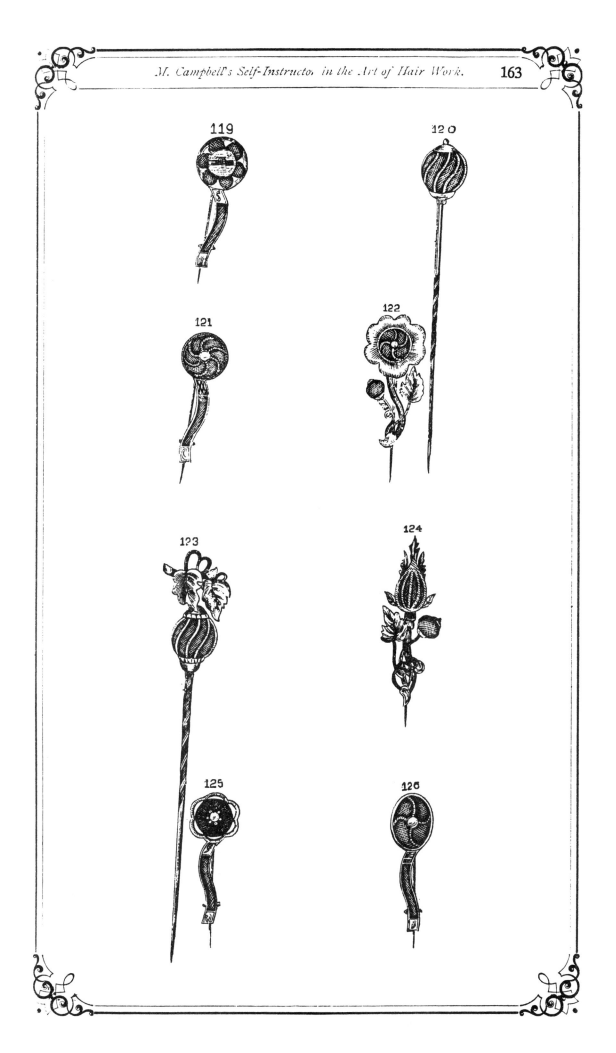

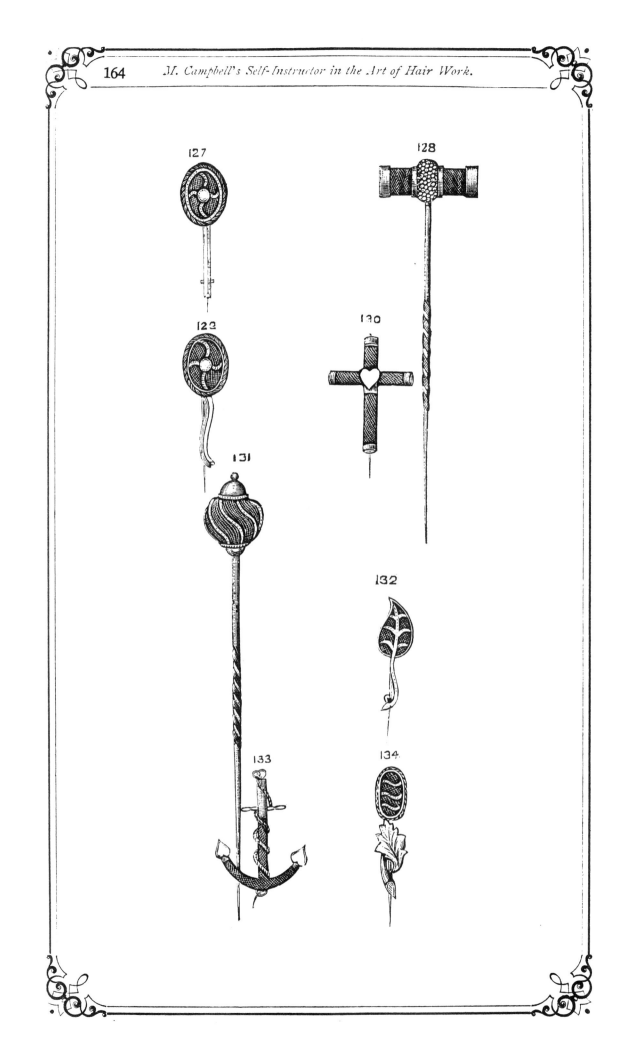

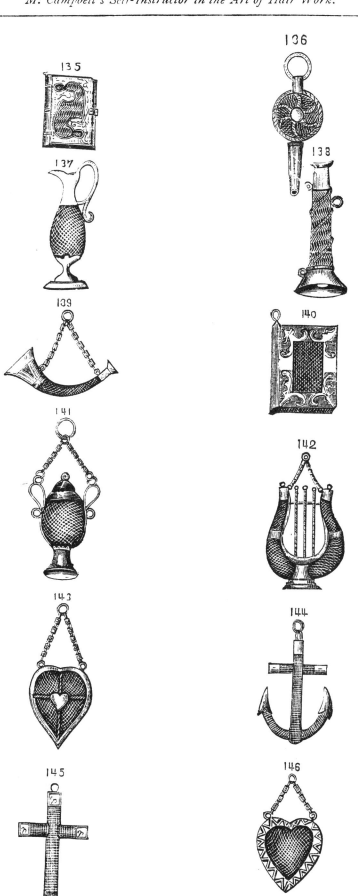

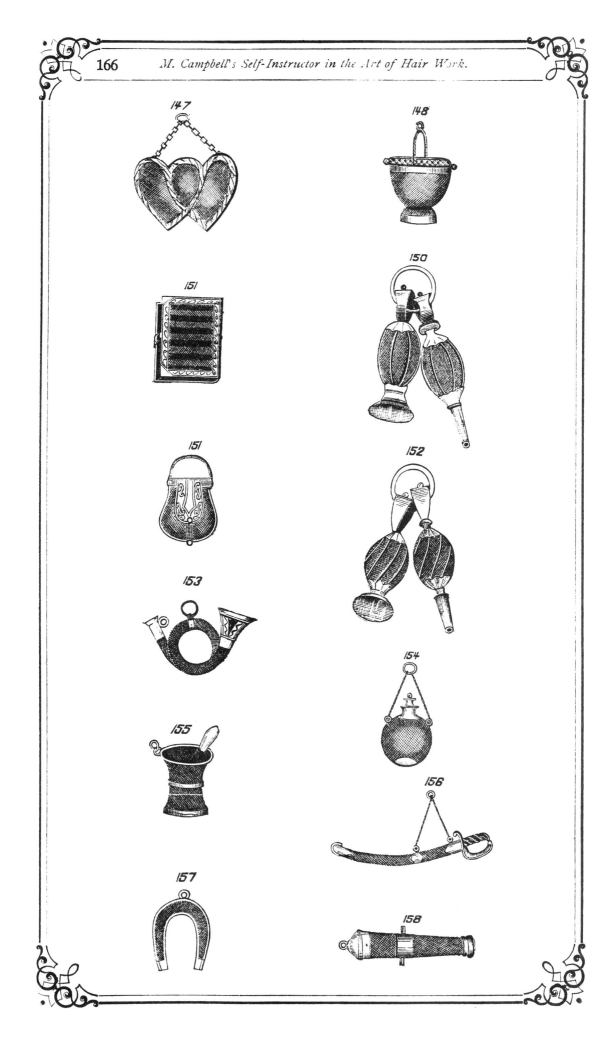

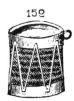

159

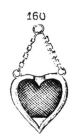

160

161

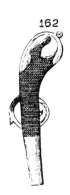

162

163

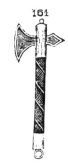

164

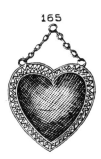

165

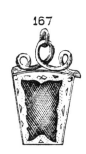

167

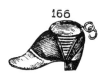

166

168

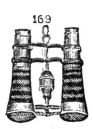

169

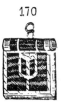

170

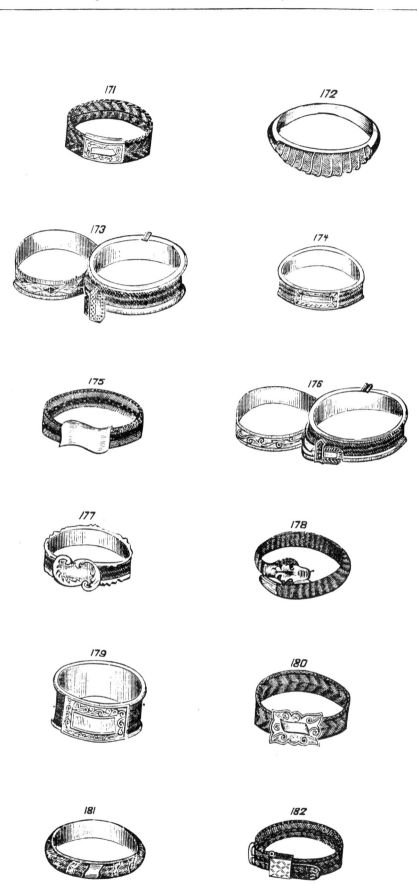

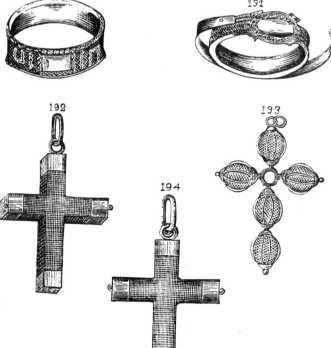

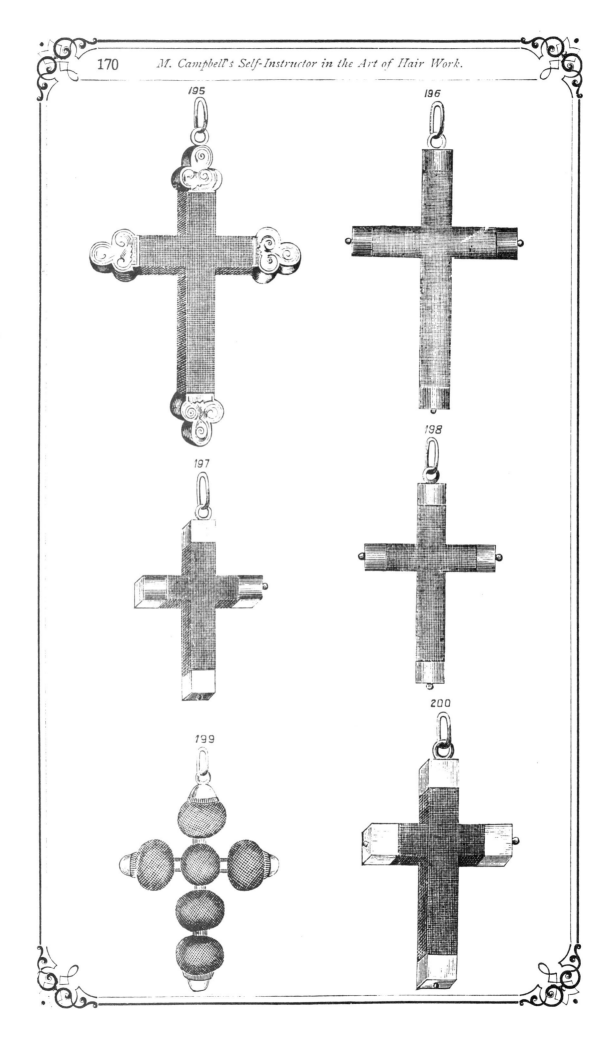

201

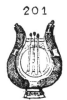

202

203

204

205

206

207

208

209

210

211

212

213

214

215

216

217

218

219

220

221

222
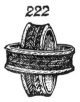

223
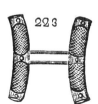

224
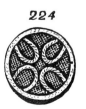

237

238

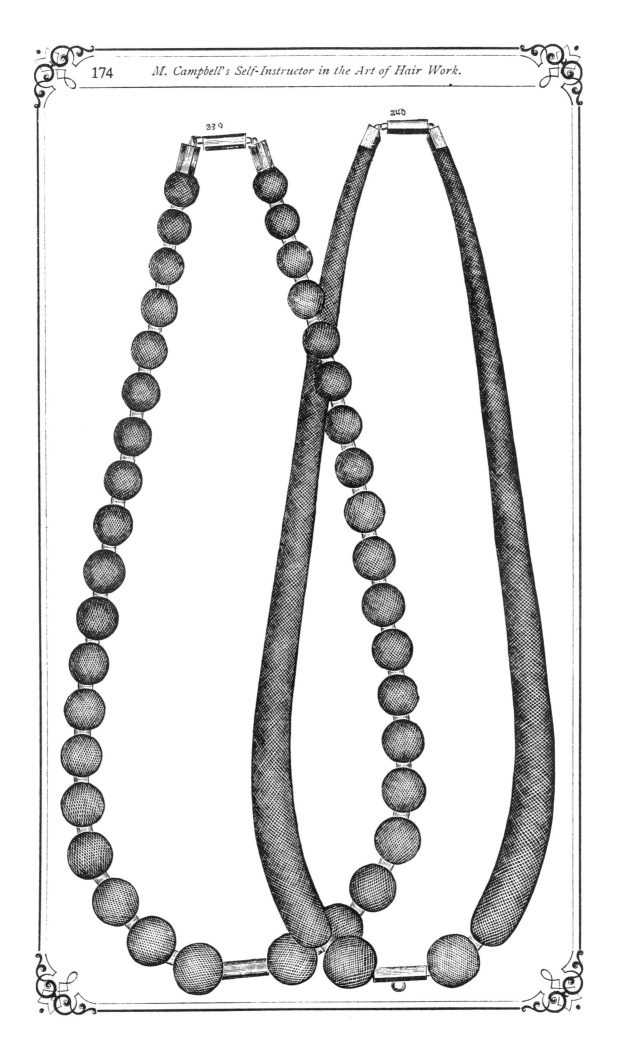

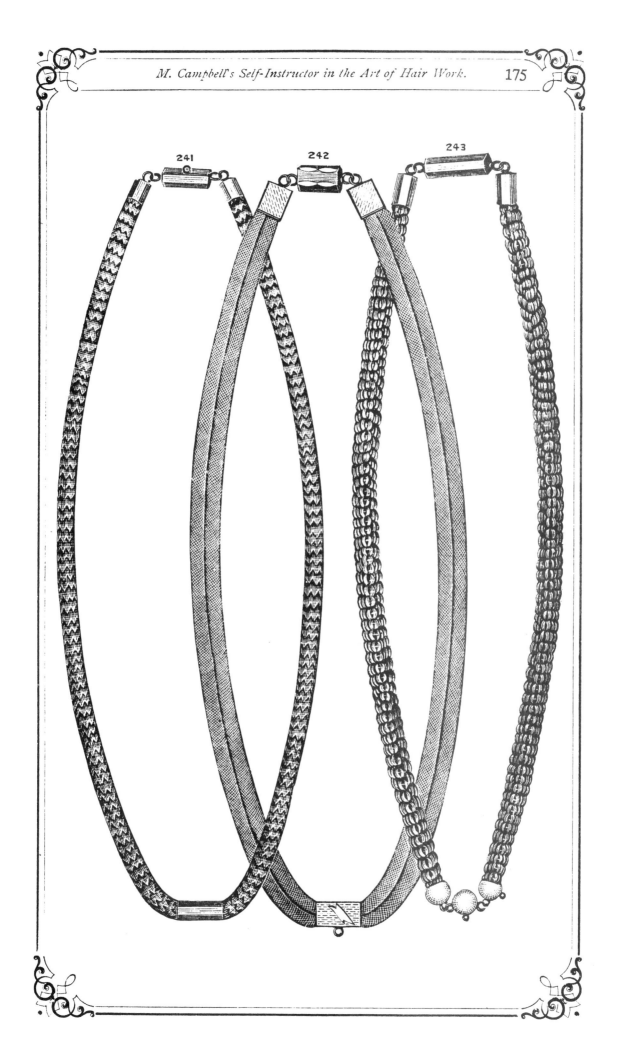

244

245

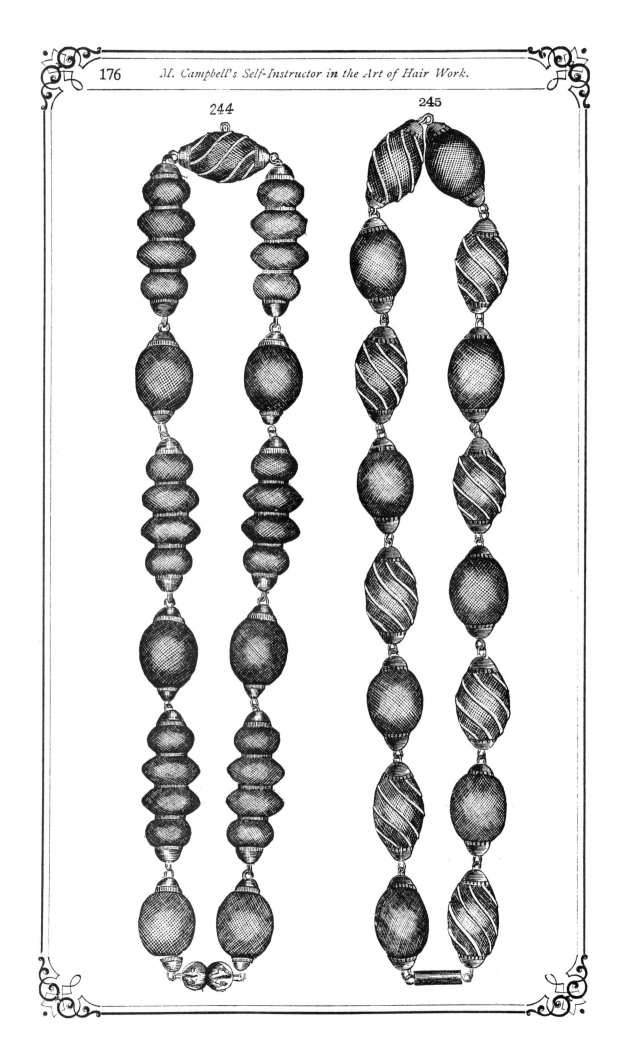

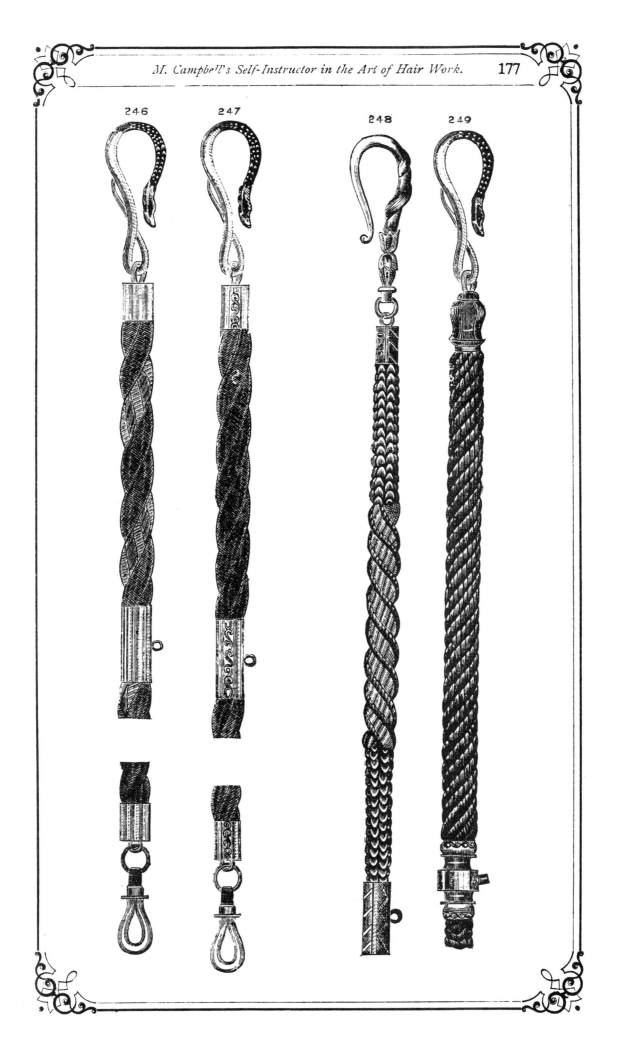

246   247   248   249

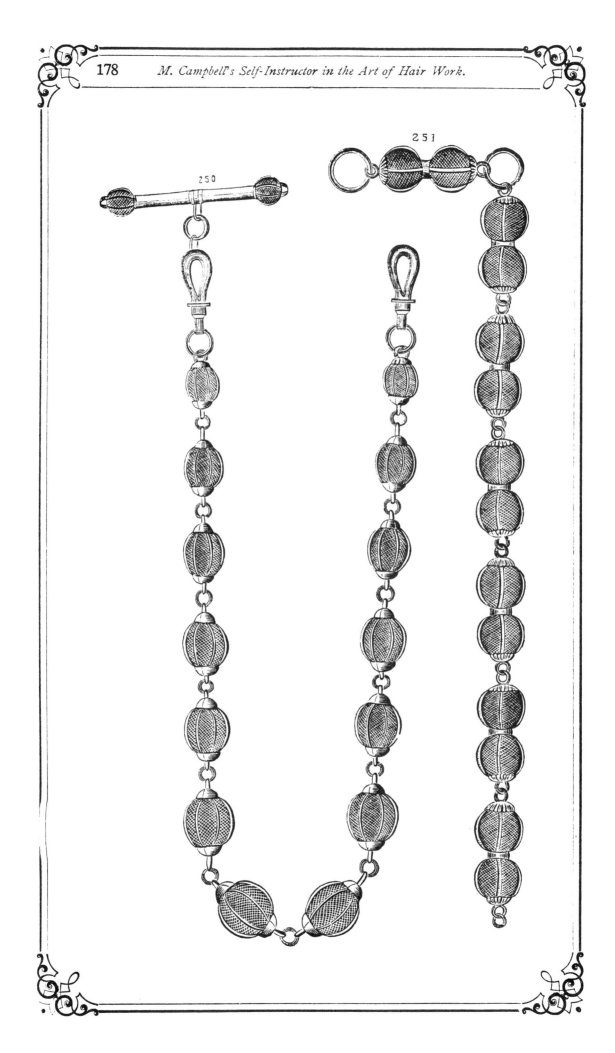

252   253   254   255

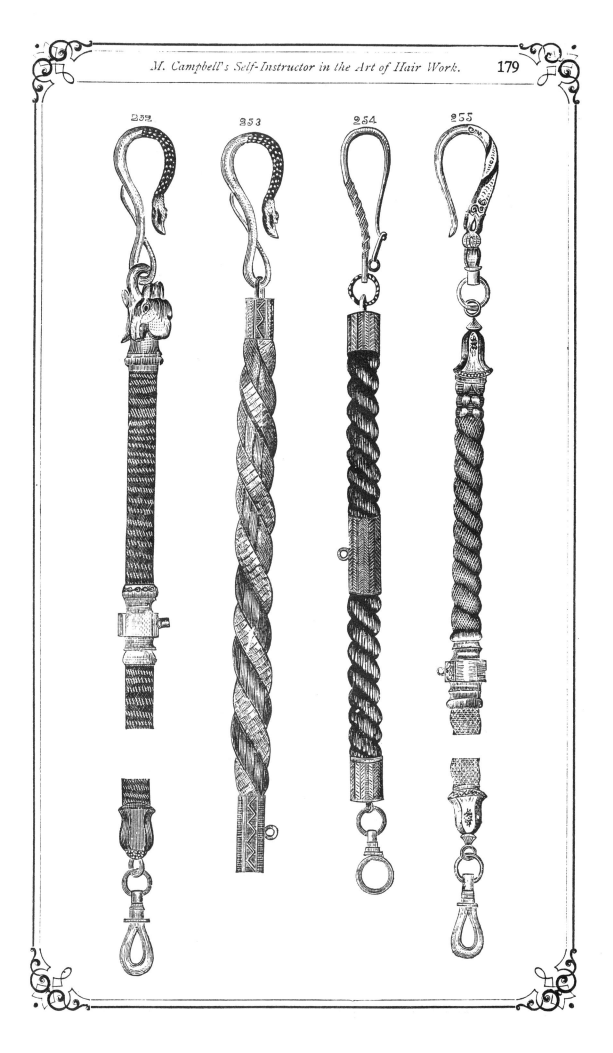

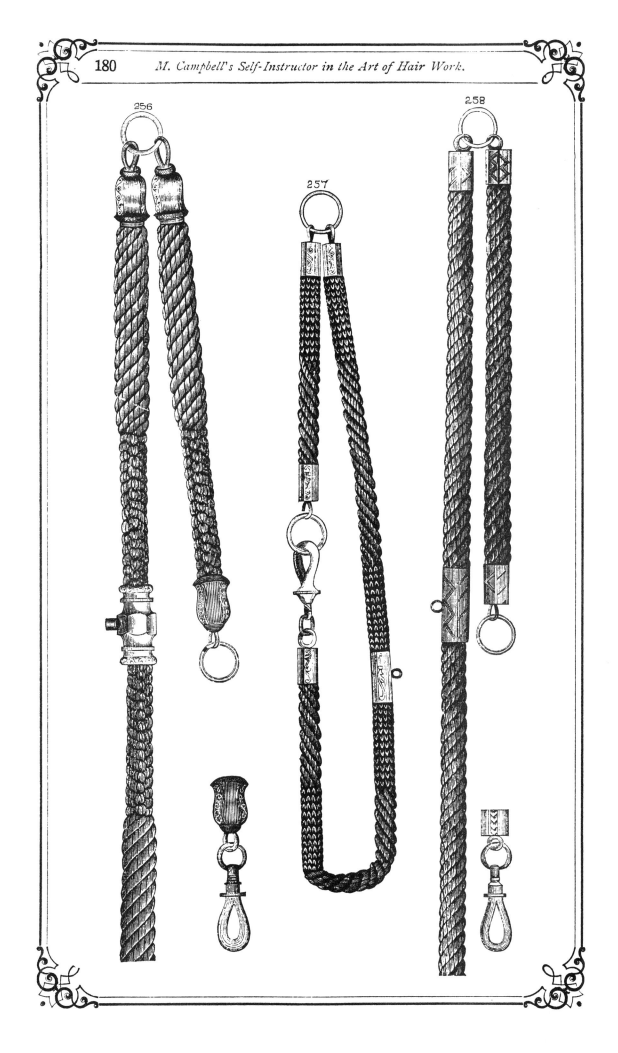

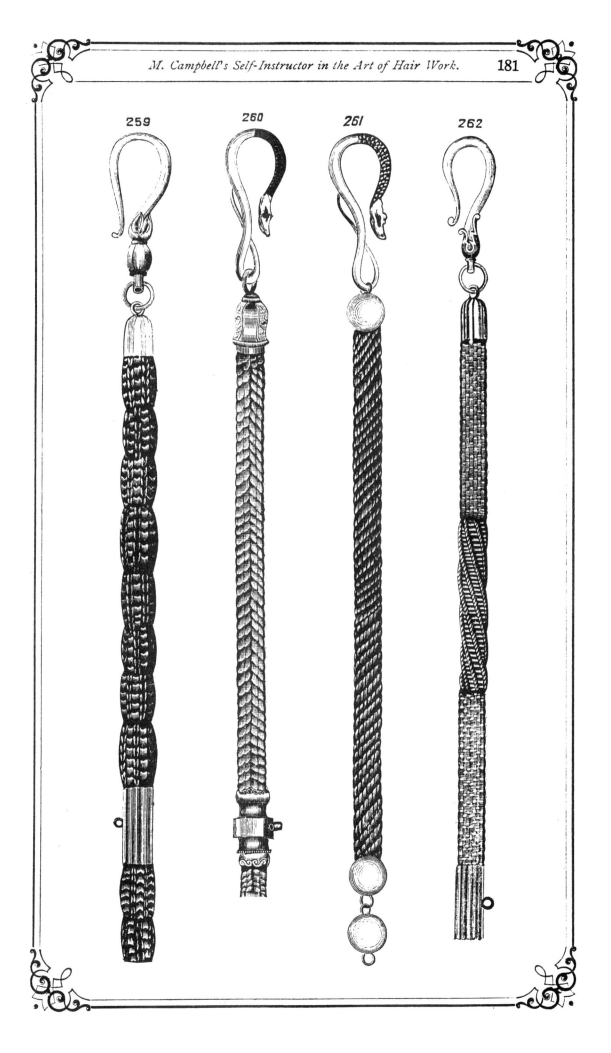

259 260 261 262

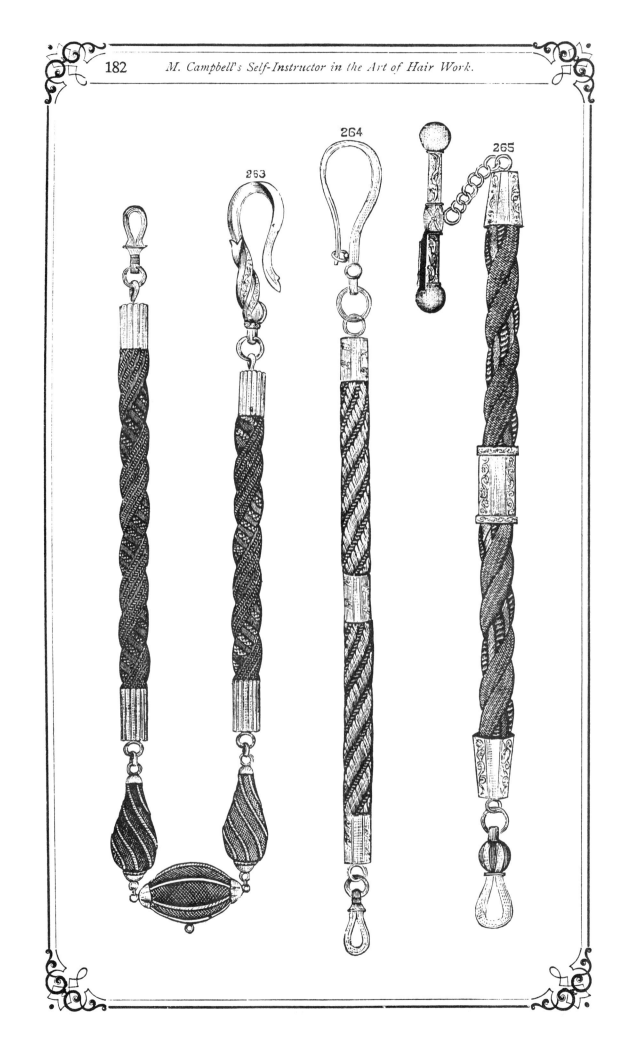

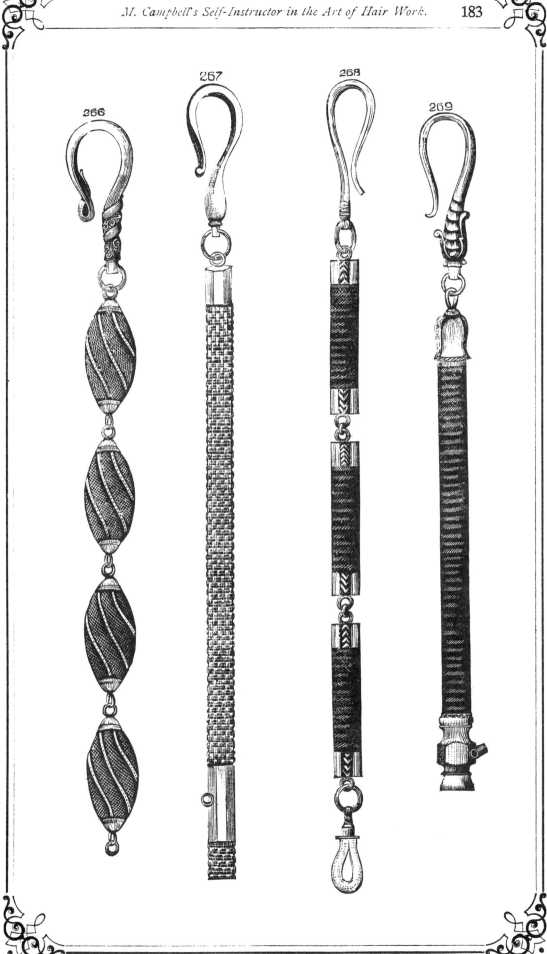

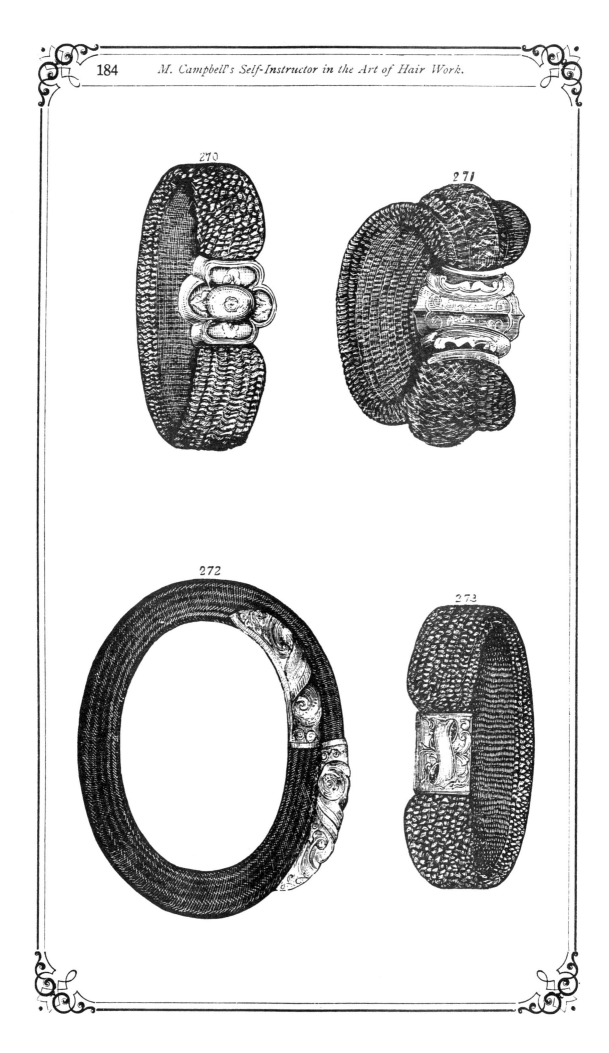

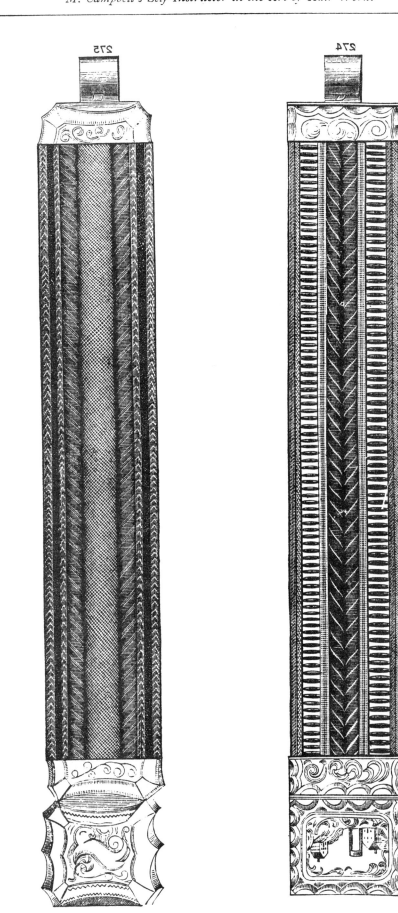

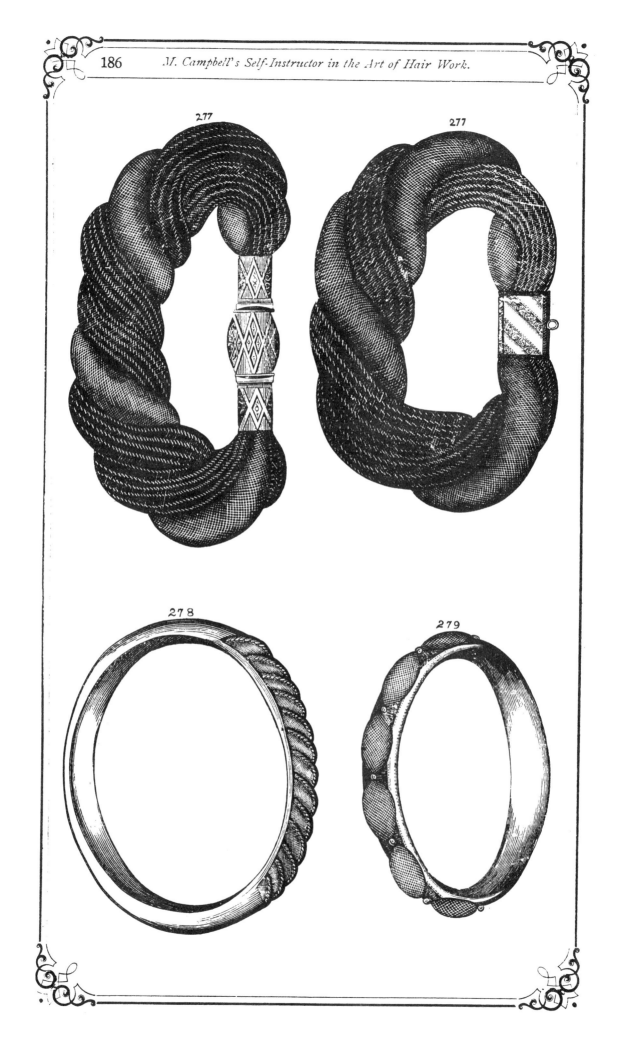

277   277

278   279

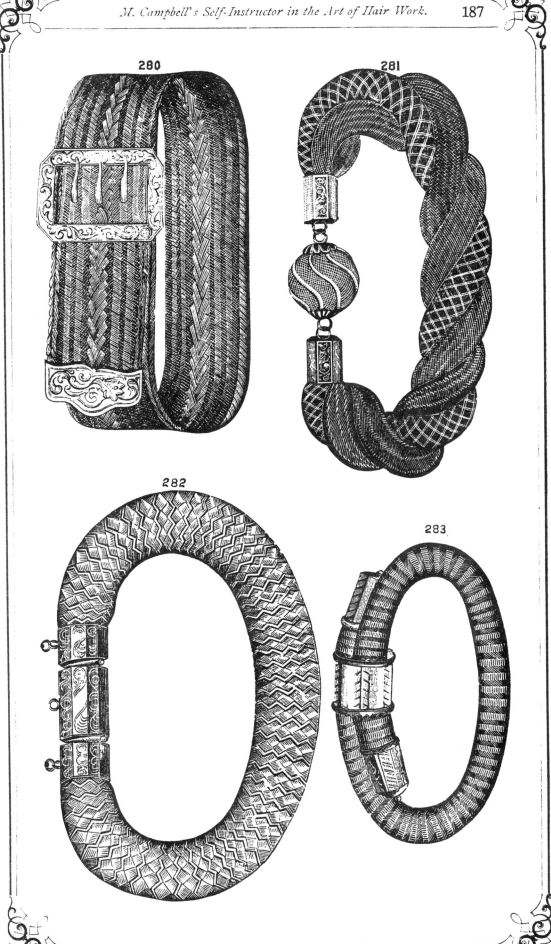

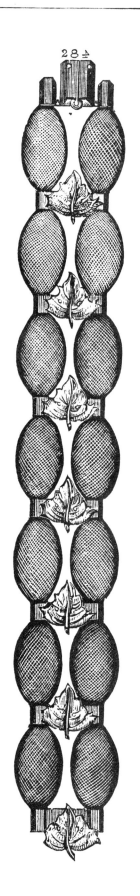

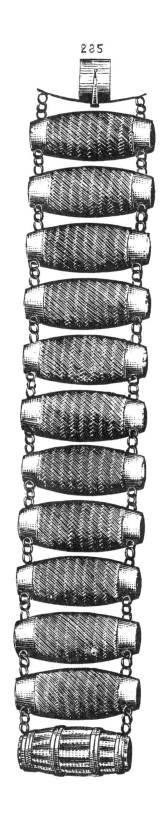

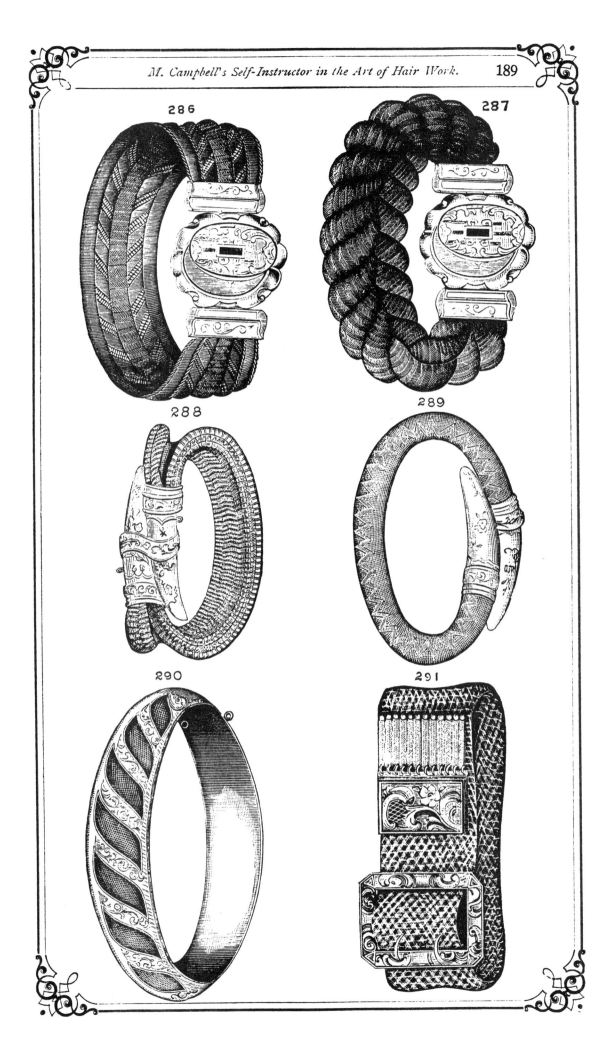

286

287

288

289

290

291

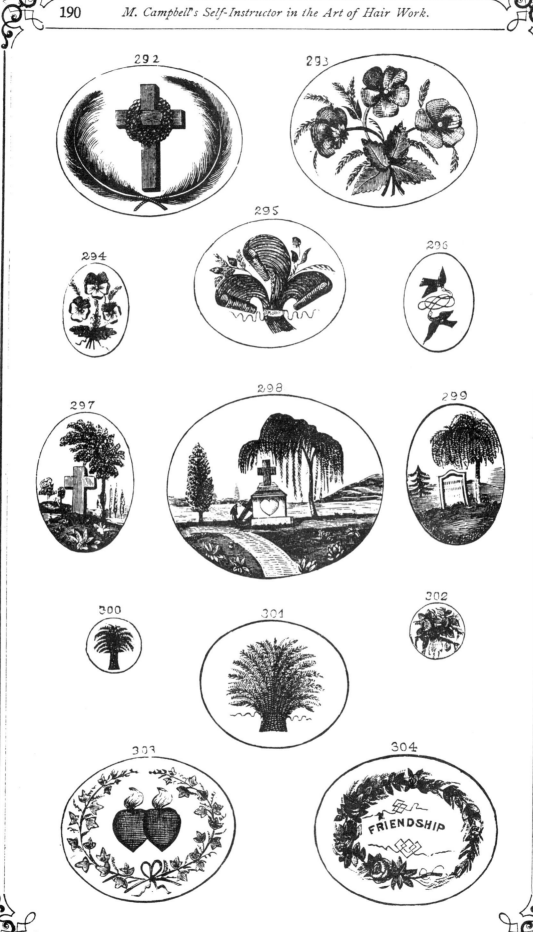

305

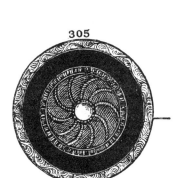

306

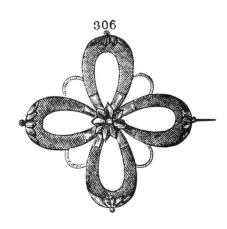

307.

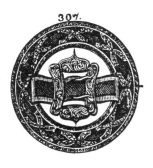

308

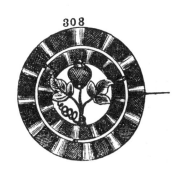

309.

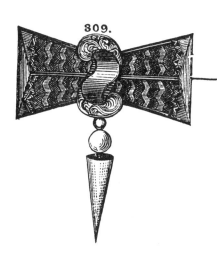

310.

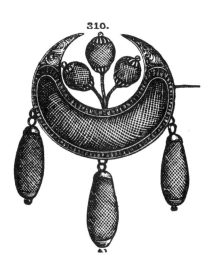

311

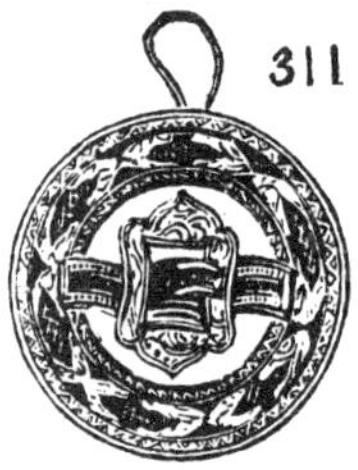

312

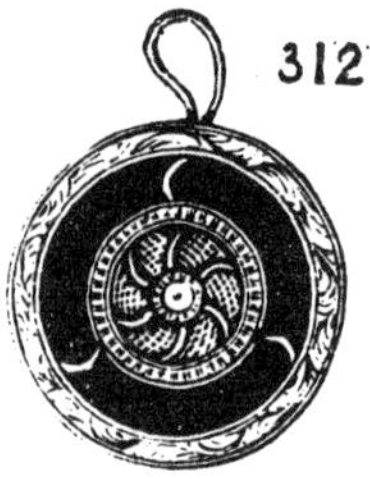

314

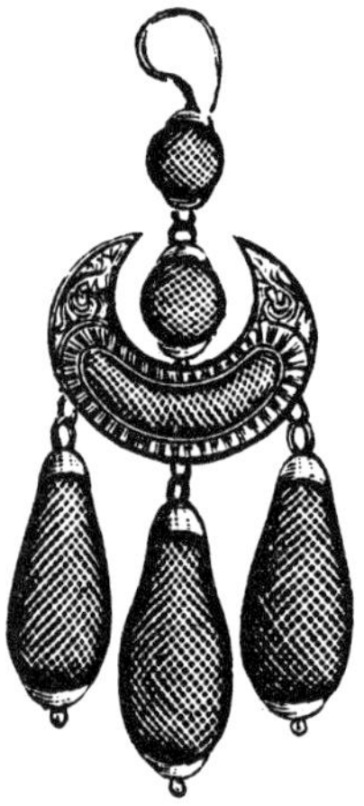

313

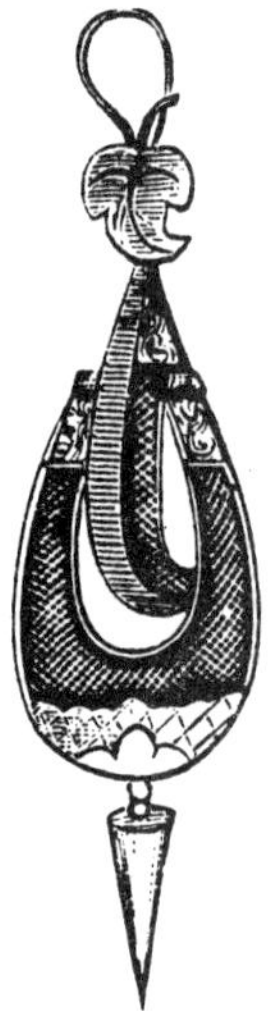

315

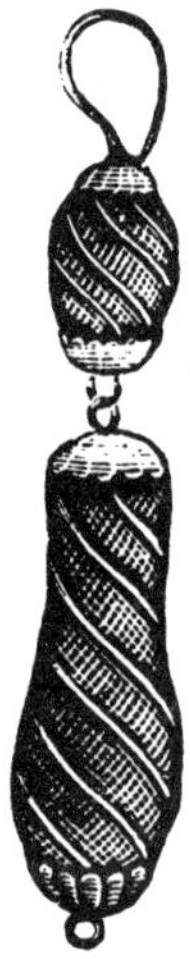

316

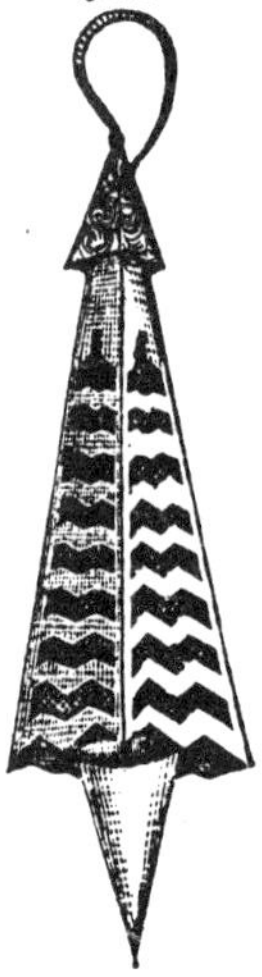

317

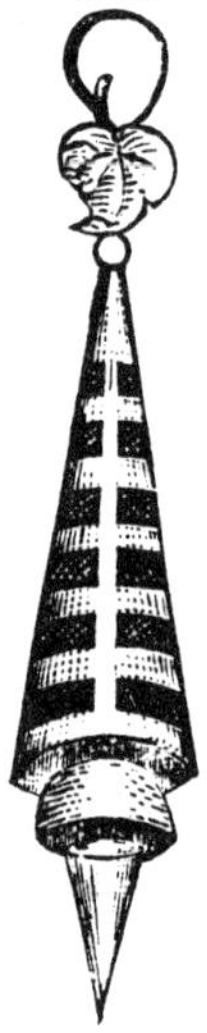

HAIR JEWELRY.

PRICE LIST.

No.	Mount's.	Compl't.	No.	Mount's.	Compl't.
1	$ 5 50	$ 8 00	52	$ 7 00	$8 00
2	3 75	6 00	53	5 00	6 00
3	3 00	5 00	54	6 50	8 00
4	5 25	8 00	55	10 00	12 00
5	4 00	7 00	56	5 00	6 00
6	4 50	7 00	57	6 00	7 00
7	6 00	10 00	58	8 00	10 00
8	5 50	8 00	59	7 00	10 00
9	11 00	15 00	60	10 00	15 00
10	10 00	12 50	61	8 00	10 00
11	6 00	8 00	62	6 00	7 00
12	5 50	8 00	63	12 50	15 00
13	8 00	10 00	64	15 00	17 50
14	6 00	8 00	65	12 50	15 00
15	4 50	6 00	66	15 00	17 50
16	9 00	12 00	67	12 50	15 00
17	7 50	10 00	68	12 50	15 00
18	6 50	8 00	69	13 00	15 00
19	12 00	15 00	70	11 00	12 50
20	9 00	12 50	71	13 00	15 00
21	7 50	10 00	72	13 00	15 00
22	10 00	12 50	73	15 00	18 00
23	8 00	10 00	74	11 00	12 50
24	7 50	10 00	75	10 00	12 50
25	10 00	15 00	76	8 00	10 00
26	12 50	15 00	77	6 50	8 00
27	4 00	7 00	78	6 50	8 00
28	4 00	8 00	79	8 50	10 00
29	10 00	12 00	80	10 00	13 00
30	10 00	12 50	81	10 00	12 50
31	15 00	17 50	82	8 00	10 00
32	15 00	17 50	83	12 00	15 00
33	12 50	15 00	84	6 00	8 00
34	12 50	15 00	85	8 00	10 00
35	12 50	15 00	86	10 00	12 50
36	12 50	15 00	87	8 00	10 00
37	13 00	15 00	88	6 50	8 00
38	11 00	12 50	89	10 00	12 00
39	13 00	15 00	90	8 00	10 00
40	13 00	15 00	91	6 00	8 00
41	15 00	18 00	92	4 50	6 00
42	11 00	12 50	93	12 50	15 00
43	10 00	12 50	94	6 00	8 00
44	8 00	10 00	95	12 00	15 00
45	6 50	8 00	96	12 00	15 00
46	6 50	8 00	97	10 00	12 50
47	8 50	10 00	98	10 00	12 50
48	10 00	12 00	99	10 00	12 00
49	4 00	5 00	100	5 00	7 00
50	4 00	5 00	101	10 00	12 00
51	4 50	6 00	102	12 50	15 00

No.	Mount's.	Compl't.	No.	Mount's.	Compl't.
103	$ 8 00	$10 00	164	$ 4 50	$5 00
104	10 00	12 00	165	5 00	6 00
105	7 00	9 00	166	4 00	4 50
106	6 00	8 00	167	6 00	7 00
107	7 00	8 00	168	4 00	4 50
108	6 00	7 00	169	7 00	8 00
109	9 00	10 00	170	6 00	7 00
110	6 00	7 00	171	1 00	1 50
111	12 00	15 00	172	4 50	5 00
112	13 00	15 00	173	11 00	12 00
113	13 00	15 00	174	3 50	4 00
114	12 00	15 00	175	1 00	1 50
115	4 50	6 00	176	9 50	10 00
116	4 00	5 00	177	5 50	6 00
117	5 00	7 00	178	3 00	4 00
118	5 00	7 00	179	6 00	7 00
119	7 00	8 00	180	1 50	2 00
120	5 00	6 00	181	6 00	7 00
121	5 00	6 00	182	2 50	3 00
122	7 00	8 00	183	6 00	7 00
123	9 00	10 00	184	4 50	5 00
124	6 00	7 00	185	6 00	7 00
125	5 00	6 00	186	4 50	5 00
126	6 00	7 00	187	7 50	8 00
127	4 50	5 00	188	5 50	6 00
128	7 00	8 00	189	9 00	10 00
129	4 50	5 00	190	11 00	12 00
130	5 00	6 00	191	9 00	10 00
131	7 00	8 00	192	3 50	5 00
132	5 50	6 00	193	8 50	10 00
133	5 00	6 00	194	3 50	5 00
134	5 50	6 00	195	10 00	15 00
135	6 00	7 00	196	5 00	8 00
136	5 50	6 00	197	4 50	7 00
137	4 00	5 00	198	4 00	6 00
138	4 25	5 00	199	4 00	6 00
139	4 25	5 00	200	6 00	10 00
140	6 00	8 00	201	10 00	12 00
141	6 00	7 00	202	12 00	15 00
142	5 00	6 00	203	8 00	10 00
143	4 00	5 00	204	6 50	8 00
144	3 00	5 00	205	4 00	5 00
145	2 50	3 50	206	10 00	12 00
146	4 00	5 00	207	8 00	10 00
147	6 50	8 00	208	10 00	12 00
148	4 00	5 00	209	6 50	8 00
149	8 00	10 00	210	12 00	13 00
150	10 00	12 00	211	8 50	10 00
151	4 25	5 00	212	9 00	10 00
152	10 00	12 00	213	8 50	10 00
153	3 50	4 50	214	10 00	12 00
154	3 50	4 00	215	8 50	10 00
155	4 00	5 00	216	6 00	7 00
156	5 25	6 00	217	13 00	15 00
157	3 50	4 00	218	13 00	15 00
158	3 50	4 50	219	8 50	10 00
159	5 00	6 00	220	8 50	10 00
160	3 50	4 00	221	7 00	8 00
161	4 00	5 00	222	10 00	12 00
162	3 50	4 00	223	7 00	8 00
163	5 00	6 00	224	8 50	10 00

No.	Mount's.	Compl't.	No.	Mount's.	Compl't.
225	$10 50	$12 00	272	$ 4 50	$8 00
226	8 50	10 00	273	4 00	6 00
227	10 50	12 00	274	9 00	12 00
228	14 00	15 00	275	9 00	12 00
229	10 00	12 00	276	7 50	10 00
230	14 00	15 00	277	3 50	6 00
231	8 50	10 00	278	18 00	20 00
232	8 50	10 00	279	18 00	20 00
233	10 00	12 00	280	17 00	20 00
234	7 50	9 00	281	9 00	12 00
235	7 50	9 00	282	12 00	15 00
236	6 75	8 00	283	9 00	12 00
237	2 25	6 00	284	16 00	20 00
238	11 00	15 00	285	30 00	40 00
239	7 00	10 00	286	9 00	12 00
240	3 50	7 00	287	9 00	14 00
241	3 50	6 00	288	4 50	6 00
242	4 50	7 00	289	4 00	7 00
243	6 00	8 00	290	18 00	20 00
244	12 00	20 00	291	22 00	25 00
245	20 00	28 00	292		6 50
246	8 00	12 00	293		6 00
247	8 00	12 00	294		4 00
248	8 00	10 00	295		5 00
249	10 00	12 00	296		4 50
250	25 00	30 00	297		5 50
251	25 00	30 00	298		8 00
252	13 00	15 00	299		6 00
253	8 00	12 00	800		2 25
254	18 00	20 00	301		4 50
255	10 00	12 00	302		2 50
256	12 00	15 00	303		7 50
257	8 00	10 00	304		6 00
258	10 00	12 00	805	18 00	20 00
259	9 50	12 00	806	13 00	15 00
260	10 00	12 00	807	23 00	25 00
261	10 25	12 00	808	15 00	17 50
262	8 00	10 00	309	22 00	25 00
263	16 00	20 00	310	12 00	15 00
264	10 00	12 00	311	23 00	25 00
265	21 00	25 00	312	18 00	20 00
266	25 00	30 00	313	23 00	25 00
267	6 00	8 00	314	12 00	15 00
268	25 00	30 00	315	15 00	18 00
269	10 00	14 00	316	22 00	25 00
270	3 50	6 00	317	18 00	20 00
271	4 00	7 00			

GODEY'S

LADY'S BOOK

AND

MAGAZINE.

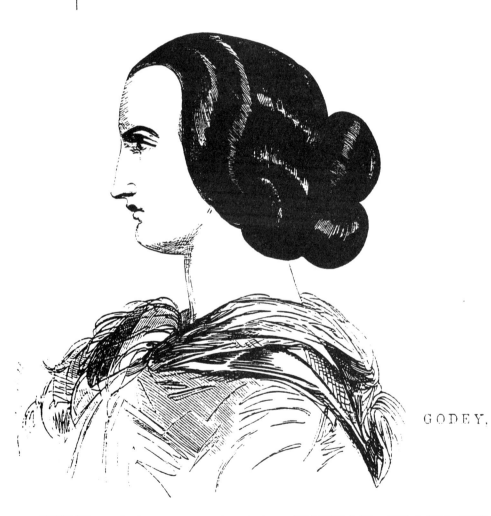

GODEY.

THE ART OF ORNAMENTAL HAIR-WORK.

Of the various employments for the fingers lately introduced among our countrywomen, none is, perhaps, more interesting than that which we are about to describe, viz., hair work; a recent importation from Germany, where it is very fashionable. Hitherto almost exclusively confined to professed manufacturers of hair trinkets, this work has now become a drawing-room occupation, as elegant and as free from all the annoyances and objections of litter, dirt, or unpleasant smells, as the much-practiced knitting, netting, and crochet can be; while a small handkerchief will at any time cover the apparatus and materials in use. By acquiring a knowledge of this art, ladies will be themselves enabled to manufacture the hair of beloved friends and relatives into bracelets, chains, rings, ear-rings, and devices, and thus insure that they do actually wear the memento they prize, and not a fabric substituted for it, as we fear has sometimes been the case.

DIRECTIONS FOR PREPARING THE HAIR.—Sort the tress, which is about to be used, into lengths, tie the ends firmly and quite straight with pack-thread, put the hair into a small saucepan with about a pint and a half of water, and a piece of soda of the size of a nut, and boil it for a quarter of an hour or twenty minutes; take it out, shake off the superfluous moisture, and hang it up to dry, but not near a fire. When it has become perfectly dry, divide it into strands containing from twenty to thirty hairs each, according to the fineness of the hair or the directions given for the pattern about to be worked. It must be observed that every hair in the strand should be of the same length, and the strands should be all, as nearly as may be, of an equal length. Knot each end of each strand, then take the requisite number of leaden weights, weighing about three quarters or half an ounce each, and affix about a quarter of a yard of pack-thread to each of them; lay them down side by side on the table, and to the other ends of the pack-thread affix the strands of hair already prepared, knotting them on with a weaver's or sailor's knot; care must be taken all this time to prevent any entanglement or derangement of the hair. The other ends of the strands must now be gathered together, firmly tied with pack-thread, and then gummed with a cement composed of equal parts of yellow wax and shell-lac melted together and well amalgamated, and then rolled into sticks for use. We now come to the table and the arrangement of the strands on it.

The accompanying cut (Fig. 1) will exemplify the directions we are now about to give. To the tied and cemented cluster of ends attach a loop of pack-thread, and hook this on to the small hook in the hole in the centre of the table; then lift each strand gently and separately off, and arrange them all smoothly and evenly round the table in the pro-

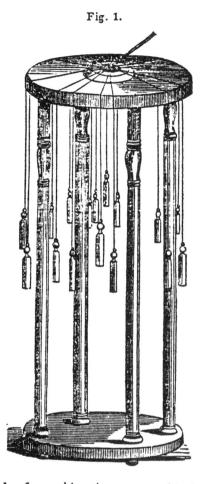

Fig. 1.

per order for working the pattern; this done, affix the balance-weight (a collection of three or four similar to those attached to the strands) to the loop in the hole, and allow it to hang down exactly in the centre of that hole; a brass tube or wire of the requisite size for the pattern about to be worked must now be placed in the centre, with one end of it resting on the hook whence the loop of pack-thread has just been taken, and the work is ready to be commenced; each strand having been first examined to see that no loose hairs hang about. When the pattern is completed, the centre or balance-weight must be detached, and then the pack-threads holding the other weights should be gathered together and cut off. Afterwards, smooth the short ends of the strands of hair on the tube and tie them tightly down to it with thread; then cut off the cemented end, and tie those parts also down in the same way. Take the tube and immerse it in scalding water, and let it simmer there, with the hair work on it, for about ten minutes; withdraw it, shake off the superfluous moisture, and hang it up to dry, not too near a fire; when thoroughly dry, the work must be gently and carefully slid off the tube, each end separately cemented with the before-mentioned composition, care being taken to gather up every hair, and the pattern will appear complete and ready to receive whatever clasp, snap, or slide it is thought proper to affix to it.

The table is very simple in its construction, and costs a mere trifle; the chief thing necessary is that every part of it should be perfectly smooth, as the least roughness or inequality would be liable to tear the hair, and thus destroy the evenness and beauty of the work. There are two varieties of the table; the first, or "ladies' table," stands about thirty-two or thirty-three inches high; the second stands nearly four feet high, and is used by the opposite sex. For our own part, we prefer the latter; for, although it may be more fatiguing to stand than to sit, more command of the work is obtained; besides, ladies' dresses, when sitting, interfere with and disturb the weights and their respective strands, and if one stands to work at the small table for even a few moments, the fatigue of stooping is very great.

We will now proceed to give some of the patterns

A PATTERN FOR A CHAIN OR GUARD. (Fig. 2.)—For this pattern, sixteen strands, each consisting of about twenty hairs, are required. These must be arranged in pairs on the circle of the table, at equal distances, and so that the opposite pairs shall be in direct lines with each other, thus: Number them with a piece

Fig. 2.

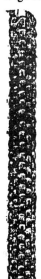

Fig. 3.

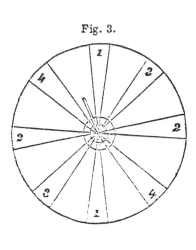

of white crayon chalk, as in the above diagram (Fig. 3), and commence working as follows: Take up the two bottom strands over figure 1, and remove them to the position of the opposite pair over the opposite figure 1, bringing back that opposite pair to the position before occupied by those just removed. Proceed then to the pair of strands over the right hand figure 2, and in the same manner lift them into the places of the strands over the opposite figure 2, and bring these latter back. Work those

over figure 3 and figure 4 in the same manner, lifting those from the right hand side over to the left, and bringing the latter back. Then recommence at figure 1, and repeat this pattern until the hair is worked up; remembering never to cross the strands, but simply lift them over gently and without jerking from one side to the other. This chain may be worked in pieces of three or four inches each, and then united with gold slides, or in only two or three portions, or in one continuous length; but this latter plan would require the hair to be longer than we can usually obtain it, namely, from fifteen to twenty inches or more in length. It should be worked on a brass wire of about the size of a No. 15 or 16 knitting needle.

A PATTERN FOR A BRACELET. (Fig. 4.)—Sixteen strands of twenty-five or thirty hairs each, according to the fineness of the hair. For this pattern the strands must be arranged in fours, and numbered thus: Take the strand which lies on figure 1, at the

Fig. 4.

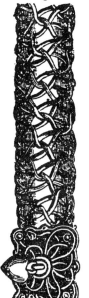

Fig. 5.

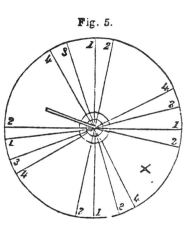

bottom of the diagram (Fig. 5), and move it towards the left, and into the place of the next figure 1 strand, lifting that and carrying it to the top of figure 1 strand, while this latter in its turn must be removed to the place of the right hand figure 1 strand, which goes to fill the vacant place of the one first lifted at the bottom. Proceed now to figure 2 of the bottom group, and work the strands numbered 2 round in the same way, and in the same direction. The next strand to be raised is figure 3 of the bottom group, and this is to be worked in the same way, but in the *opposite* direction, viz., towards the right and into the place of strand 3 on the right of the ×, which in its turn goes to the top, and the top one to the left, while that from the left hand group comes to the vacant figure 3 at the bottom. Figure 4 is worked in the same way and direction as the threes; then recommence at 1.

The point to be observed is to move the ones and twos towards the left, and the threes and fours towards the right; always beginning from the bottom group. This pattern should be worked on a brass tube of the thickness of an ordinary lead pencil, or rather larger; and it looks very well over another and closer plait—such, for instance, as the one we first described. Each must then be worked separately, and when finished and perfectly dry, the smaller one should be passed through the larger, and the ends of the two cemented firmly together. For such purpose, we should advise that the Fig. 2 pattern should be worked on a larger wire, perhaps of the size of a No. 10 knitting needle.

CHAIN OR GUARD PATTERN. (Fig. 6.) — Ten strands only, of about twenty hairs each, are required for this. They must be arranged thus: Take figure 1 from the bottom, and move it round in the direction

Fig. 6.

Fig. 7.

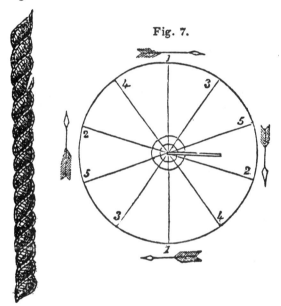

pointed out by the arrows into the place of figure 1 at the top, bringing that round and down to the bottom; so on with the twos, threes, fours, and fives, always working in the direction pointed out—namely, lifting the right hand strand into the place of the left, and that round to the right: they should be lifted round, and not crossed over. A wire about the size of a No. 15 knitting needle will do best to work this on. Bear in mind that the strands are to be worked in the order in which they are numbered.

A very pretty bracelet may be made with this pattern by increasing the size of the strands (putting from thirty to thirty-five hairs in each), and working on a tube of the size of a No. 6 knitting needle.

Three lengths of the pattern must then be made, and twisted together so as to form a kind of rope or cable, and firmly cemented together at the ends.

A BRACELET PATTERN. (Fig. 8.)—Thirty-two strands, of from twenty to thirty hairs each, and arranged in groups of fours, as evenly as possible, are needed for this pattern, which may be worked on a tube of the same size ordered for Fig. 4 pattern, or on a flat brass mesh about half or three-quarters of an inch in breadth, or on a mould large at one end and diminishing towards the other. In this latter form, it constitutes the fashionable snake bracelet.

A cross must be made with crayon chalk to indicate where the pattern always commences; and

Fig. 8.

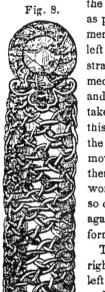

the strands must be kept as much as possible in their places. Commence thus, working towards the left: Take the outside right hand strand of the first group of four immediately on the left of the cross, and pass it over the one next to it; take the outside left hand strand of this same group, and pass it over the two next to it; repeat these movements with this group, and then proceed to the next four, and work them in the same way; and so on all round the table, until you again come to the cross. This forms the first part of the plait.

Then take two strands from the right of the cross and two from the left of it, to form the group of four, and re-arrange the fours all round, taking the outside twos of each neighboring set to form the fresh grouping. Begin as before with the four immediately on the left of the cross; take the two middle strands, and pass them over the outside ones, and then under them, and so into the middle again; cross the left hand middle strand over the right hand one, then pass the right hand outside strand over the two middle ones, and then the left hand outside strand over the three others; proceed to the next group of four and work them in the same way, and so on all round the board. The pattern is now complete; the strands must be restored to their original places and groups, and we recommence with the first part of the plait.

In working this pattern, great care must be observed in the altering and restoring the arrangement of the strands in their several groups at each change of the plait. The opposite groups must also be kept as much as possible in parallel lines, as the symmetry of the work depends on attention to these niceties.

.... *Godey's Lady's* 1850

No. 7.—Four-Ribbed Spiral Chain Plait.

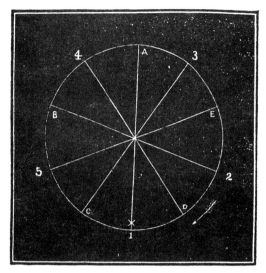

Move the opposite strands each half way round, simultaneously, in the direction of the arrow, taking them in their numerical order.

It will be observed that, to avoid confusion from duplicate numbers, the strand opposite to 1 is called A, to 2 B, to 3 C, and so on.

It is immaterial with which hand the strands are taken up, provided that they are moved in the direction of the arrow. The worker will, perhaps, find it easiest to take up 3 and 4 with the right hand, and 5, 1, and 2 with the left.

Thus, take up 1 with the left and A with the right hand; pass 1 over C 5, B, and 4, and lay it down at A; and at the same time pass A over 3 E, 2, and D, and lay it down at 1.

Next, take 2 with the left, and B with the right; pass 2 over D 1 C 5, and lay it down at B; and at the same time pass B over 4 A 3 E, and lay it down at 2.

    Then, 3 (right) o. E 2, D 1, to C.
      and C (left) o. 5 B, 4 A, to 3.
    Then, 4 (right) o. A 3, E 2, to D.
      and D (left) o. 1 C, 5 B, to 4.
    Lastly, 5 (left) o. B 4, A 3, to E.
      and E (right) o. 2 D, 1 C, to 5.

There is a much easier way of doing this plait, but we cannot recommend it, because it is more tedious. It is this:—

Take the letters in the right hand and the figures in the left, and turn the table partly round between each movement of the strands, so that when you are moving 2 and B they shall be in front of you, as 1 and A were when you proceeded to change them over. When 2 and B have changed places, turn the table till 3 and C are in front of you, and so on with the rest.

Though this method is more simple, it will take just twice as long to do a piece of work as the other plan.

This plait has not sufficient firmness to enable it to fly back to its proper form after having been stretched out, because the act of pulling it out alters the arrangement of the stitches in the work, in which altered arrangement the piece of work will remain. In order to prevent this, a piece of elastic of the same or nearly the same size as the mould must be put into the piece of work as soon as the mould has been removed; when this has been fastened to the work at each end, the elasticity of the work may be tried, but not before. The elastic inside will prevent any alteration in its form.

The annexed figure of this plait shows it to have four spiral ridges.

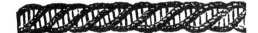

On comparing it with the four-ribbed spiral plait No. 4, it will be found to differ materially from it.

No. 8.—Close Spiral Chain Plait.

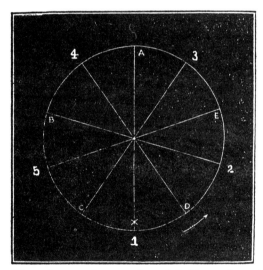

Move the opposite strands each half round simultaneously to the right, taking them in their numerical order.

This plait is much like No. 4; but a very different effect is produced by moving all the strands *to the right* (instead of to the left, as in No. 4); that is, 1 must pass over D, 2, E, and 3, while A is passing over 4, B, 5, and C, and so with the rest.

If the more tedious way of moving the table round be adopted, it is very easy to remember to take the letters in the left hand and the figures in the right.

A very similar but looser plait is made by stretching out No. 4, without putting elastic inside. The annexed cut gives a representa-

tion of the plait so made, by which plan the chain possesses very little elasticity.

To make an elastic chain like this, rule No. 8 must be followed, and elastic put into the work.

No. 9.—Two-ribbed, Double-Ribbed Spiral Chain Plait.

Move the opposite strands each half round simultaneously, alternately to the right and to the left, taking them up in their numerical order.

THIS plait is essentially the same as the two previous plaits, the only difference (nevertheless an important one in the resulting work) being, that instead of all the strands being moved in one direction, every other pair is moved half round in the opposite direction, thus : 1 and A go to the right, 2 and B to the left, 3 and C to the right, 4 and D to the left, 5 and E to the right, 1 and A to the left (not to the right this time), and so on.

This at first appears to be a very troublesome plait to work, but such is not the case if a little attention be given to it. The simplest and least confusing way of doing it is to turn the table at each move, and to say to yourself while doing it, "1 right, 2 left, 3 right, 4 left, 5 right, A left, B right, C left, D right, E left, 1 right," e c., and to remember to take the strand so numbered with the hand so mentioned, that is, 1 with the right hand, 2 with the left, and so on alternately. By attending to this, there is no need to think about the direction in which the strand is to be moved, because if 1 *be taken in the right hand* and A in the left, you would naturally make them change places by passing 1 over D, 2, E, and 3, and A over 4, B, 5, and C; in other words, you would move both strands round *to the right*.

This is a favorite chain pattern, especially when made with large strands and a small mould. Most of the receipts given for Nos. 7 and 8 will do equally well for this plait.

No. 10.—Thin Ring Plait.

Take A up in the left hand, and pass it over the pair of strands marked 4, under the pair 5, and over the pair 6.

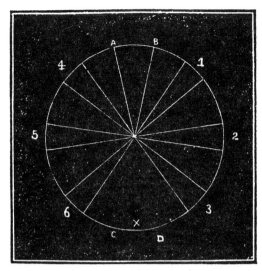

A o. 4, u. 5, o. 6, to C;
B o. 1, u. 2, o. 3, to D;
C o. D.   Rearrange.

At the same time take B up in the right hand, and pass it over the pair 1, under the pair 2, and under the pair 3.

A and B will then respectively have come to the points C and D ; now pass A over B, or rather C over D, and lay them down.

The strands must now be arranged by taking the upper strand of the pair 4 for A, and the upper strand of the pair 1 for B. In like manner pass up one from the pair 5 to complete the pair 4, and one from 6 to complete the pair 5. The strand at C then goes to make up the pair 6 ; and when a corresponding alteration has been made on the other side of the table, the rearrangement is finished. The plait may then be commenced again.

Care must be taken to keep the strands always following each other, and on no account must they be allowed to get out of order, or to cross another except where it is directed.

Although the diagram only shows fourteen strands, the plait may be worked with any number, provided that two strands are laid out for A and B, and the rest are arranged in pairs, of which there should be an equal number on each side. Should there be an uneven number, say seventeen strands, two of the additional strands must be put on one side and one on the other, the latter being considered in the light of an additional pair, under which A or B must be moved before it reaches C or D. The fact of there being eight strands on one side of the table and nine on the other will not render the work unsightly.

Where it is required to put a piece of hairwork around the outside of a gold ring, this plait will be found to be more fit for the purpose than any other.

An important recommendation which this plait has should be mentioned. It uses up hair more economically than any other; that is to say, a pretty effect is produced by this plait with less hair than by any other plait.

No mould is required. The strands should have unusually heavy bobbins put upon them, and the balance should be half the weight of the sum of the weights of the bobbins, and should hang by a piece of tape.

In order to boil the work, it must be stretched out to its full length, pinned in that condition upon a piece of cork or soft wood, and thus boiled and dried.

No. 11.—THICK RING PLAIT.

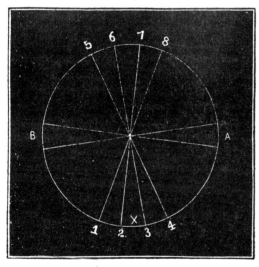

To left, 1 and 2 > 5 and 6, which take back;
To right, 3 and 4 > 7 and 8, which take back;
A > B, which take back.

In moving 1, 2, 5, and 6 to their respective places, keep them always on the left side of the mould; and keep 3, 4, 7, and 8 always to the right. The pair at A are to pass one on each side of the mould, as also the pair at B.

This plait makes a nice ring, without requiring a gold frame.

It is sufficient to unite the two ends of a piece of work, of the proper length, with a little piece of flat gold tube.

The four strands at A and B should always have fewer hairs in them than the others.

No. 12.—ROUND CHAIN PLAIT.

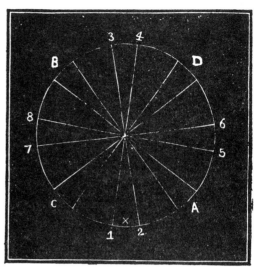

1 and 2 > 3 and 4, which take back;
5 and 6 > 7 and 8, which take back;
A > B, which take back;
C > D, which take back.

This plait is the same as No. 2, only done with 16 instead of 8 strands. It is, therefore, unnecessary to give any further description of it than is contained in the above rule.

No. 13.—SNAKE PLAIT.

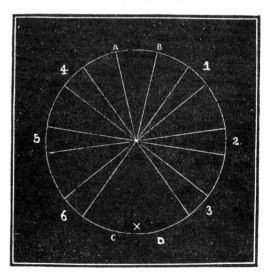

B o. A, u. 4, o. 5, u. 6, to C;
A u. 1, o. 2, u. 3, to D;
C. o. D.   Re-arrange.

The principle upon which this plait is worked is the same as that of the ring plait, No. 10. It differs from it, however, in two important points: first, it is always worked upon a mould; secondly, the plait is commenced by crossing B over A, which is not the case in the ring plait.

These dissimilarities are not likely to puzzle the beginner at all, since the presence of the mould will always remind the worker that it is necessary to cross the strands before beginning the principal part of the work.

This plait presents a peculiarity which we do not know of in any other. It is this: After finishing it off, and before boiling it, the work must be *taken off the mould*, stretched and pulled about between the fingers gently, and then slipped carefully on to the mould again; after which it is boiled. Unless this is done, the work will be too close on one side and too loose on the other.

There are other ways of working this plait.

No. 14.—Whip Plait.

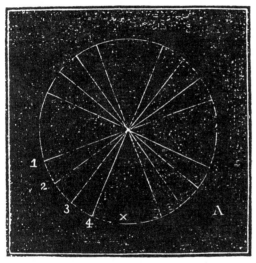

3 *o.* 2,
1 *o.* 2; 3 *o.* 4,   } 1st round to left,
3 *o.* 2.   } 2d round to right.

In order to make the explanation as simple as possible, we will suppose that you have on your table 16 strands of 20 hairs each, with 2 oz. bobbins attached to each, a balance of 8 oz., and No. 10 mould. The strands are arranged as shown on the diagram, and everything is ready for the commencement of the plaiting.

First, bring the X on the table close to you. Next, observe in which direction the first round is to be worked. In this case it is *to the left;* consequently, the group immediately on the *left* of the X is to be worked first, then the group to the left of that, and so on round the table until all the groups have been worked once, and the worker has arrived at the X again.

The plaiting of each of these groups is thus

done: 1*st*, put 3 over 2; 2*d*, put 1 over 2, and 3 over 4; 3*d*, put 3 over 2. In order that the beginner may know whether the plaiting has been correctly done, we may say that the strands which were originally called 1, 2, 3, 4 now stand in the order of 3, 4, 1, 2; nevertheless, they must not be thought of as 3, 4, 1, 2, but must be regarded in their new capacity of 1, 2, 3, 4 for any further work.

We will now conclude that this plait has been correctly worked with all the four groups, beginning with the one numbered 1, 2, 3, 4, and finishing with the one on the right of the X, the table being turned partly round to bring each group in front as it was required. Before the plaiting can be proceeded with, the whole of the strands must be arranged into fresh groups of 4; these new groups are to be made by taking a pair from each of the existing groups, and laying them down side by side, without crossing them, as shown in diagram B.

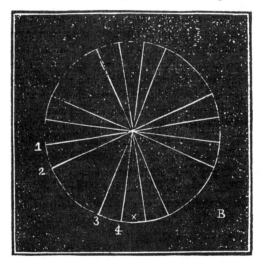

Thus, 3 and 4 of the first group on the left of the X are added to 1 and 2 of the first group on its right, and a fresh group of 4 is thus formed at the X. A fresh group should then be made opposite to it in a similar way, while the remaining 4 strands on each side will make 2 more groups at right angles to the others.

The plaiting is proceeded with by doing the *second round to the right;* that is, the group at the X is plaited first, then the group to the right, then the next group on its right, and so on till all the groups have been worked. After this the original groups are formed again, as shown on diagram A, and the plaiting of the first round is commenced again; in short, the same plait is worked in every round. The rounds are worked alternately to the left and right, and the strands are regrouped between each round, until the hair is all used up.

The result is exhibited in the accompanying figure.

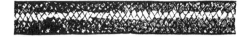

No. 15.—OPEN PLAIT.

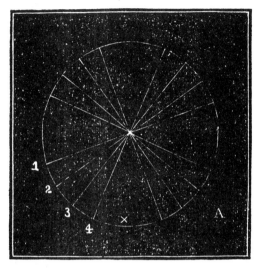

3 o. 2.
1 o. 2; 3 o. 4.   } 1st round to left.
3 o. 2.
1 o. 2; 3 o. 4.   } 2d round to right.

On comparing this rule with that for the close plait in the last number, it will be observed that the only difference consists in putting 1 over 2 and 3 over 4 at the last. With this simple exception the mode of plaiting is precisely the same, as are also the directions of the rounds and the method of regrouping. It is, therefore, unnecessary to explain it any further.

The engraving below shows what a very different effect is produced by this slight alteration in the plait.

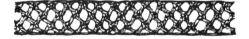

No. 16.—WAVY PLAIT.

(*Same Diagram as No. 15.*)

1st round to left.
2 u. 3, o. 4.
1 o. 2 and 3.

2d round to right.
2 o. 3, u. 4.
1 u. 2 and 3.

This plait differs from the two preceding, in the strands being moved differently in the round to the right to what they are in the round to the left: in other words, this plait is a combination of two plaits worked alternately.

After having done many pieces of this plait, I found it more easy to remember in the following form:—

to left,   3 o. 2,
             2 and 4 u. 1 and 3.
to right,   2 o. 3,
             1 and 3 u, 2 and 4.

In working round to the left I turned 3 o. 2 with the left hand, raised up 1 and 3 with the right hand, and with the left passed 2 and 4 under them; in working round to the right I turned 2 o. 3 with the right hand, and held up 2 and 4 with the left hand, while the right hand moved 1 and 3 under them.

The annexed figure shows the mode in which the strands cross each other; but an engraving cannot represent the beautifully glossy and wavy appearance of this plait.

No. 17.—BROOCH PLAIT.

(*Same Diagram as No. 15.*)

3 o. 2, and 1,   } 1st round to left.
4 u. 3 o. 4.   } 2d round to right.
1 o. 2; 3 o. 4.

There is nothing in this rule which needs explanation, the same plait being repeated in every round.

It is called the Brooch plait from its being generally preferred to any other for the bows of brooches; when bent or twisted it always retains its round form, and does not become flat at the bend as most other hollow pieces of hair-work do.

It is rather a tedious plait to do, nevertheless it well repays for the time spent upon it.

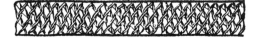

THE ART OF ORNAMENTAL HAIR-WORK.

WE come now to a different set of plaits from any that have gone before ; and as they are all worked more or less upon one common principle, viz., in groups of four strands at a time, we think it best to take the simplest of them (the common Close Plait) first, and to describe the working of it very fully. The beginner should practise this frequently before proceeding with any of the others, because, when once the principle of working it is clearly understood. the cause of any accidental errors in working any of the others, subsequently, will then be readily perceived and as easily avoided in future ; while, on the other hand, if any of the others are attempted too soon, mistakes are very likely to occur, to the disappointment of the worker, disappointment mixed with much annoyance, from not knowing how to rectify the mistakes.

From these plaits being worked in groups of 4 strands at a time, it becomes necessary to use some number of strands which will divide by 4 without a remainder, such as 16, 24, 32, 40, 48, 64, 80, or 96. We mention these numbers because hairworkers find it better to use them than such numbers as 12, 28, 36, etc.

The diagrams, for the sake of simplicity, represent only 16 strands, arranged in 4 groups of 4 strands each. If any larger number of strands—for instance, 32—are to be used for the work, they must be arranged in 8 groups, at even distances apart, taking care that each group is always kept in a line with the opposite group.

As each group is to be worked, the table must be turned so as to bring that group nearest to you. Each group is numbered, or supposed to be numbered, 1, 2, 3, 4, *from the left* to the right, as shown in diagram A.

The rules are divided into short lines, the instructions contained in each line referring to the condition of the table, or, rather, the arrangement of the group at a particular time, for the arrangements vary after every line has been worked.

Thus, "3 o. 2, 1 o. 2," means that the strands which are now numbered 1, 2, 3, 4, should be altered first to 1, 3, 2, 4, by putting 3 over 2, and next to 3, 2, 1, 4, by putting 1 over 2. To repeat,

3 o. 2, 1 o. 2,
means to alter 1, 2, 3, 4 to 3, 2, 1, **4.**
But if the rule had been written,
3 o. 2,
1 o. 2,

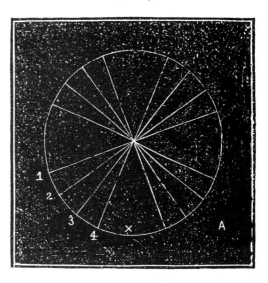

it would mean that 1, 2, 3, 4 should be ultimately changed to 2, 1, 3, 4. The reason of this is as follows : The first line directs you to put 3 over 2 ; by doing so you alter the strands from 1, 2, 3, 4 to 1, 3, 2, 4. As there are no further instructions in this line, you take your hands away from the table, and see what the next line directs. It is, that you are to put 1 over 2. You must completely forget what you have previously done, and must look at the strands in their present order, and think of them as 1, 2, 3, 4 (not 1, 3, 2, 4). Then, when you comply with the directions in the second line, you alter 1, 2, 3, 4 into 2, 1, 3, 4 ; and, if any other line were to follow, you must again regard the strands before you as 1, 2, 3, 4. In short, every line of the rule alters the original order of the strands ; but, before working out a fresh line, the strands, as they then lie, are to be considered as numbered 1, 2, 3, 4, from the left.

MANUFACTURING DEPARTMENT.

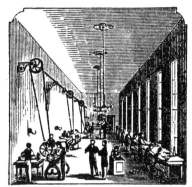

GOLD JEWELRY MANUFACTORY.

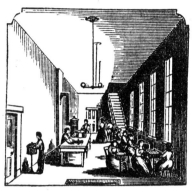

HAIR BRAIDING ROOMS.

I manufacture and sell, at WHOLESALE and RETAIL,

HAIR JEWELRY

—AND—

Gold Mountings for Hair Jewelry,

OF EVERY PATTERN AND DEVICE,

To suit the fancy of my patrons. I have given years of study and practical experience to this branch of my business, and have so perfected and enlarged my MANUFACTURING FACILITIES as to feel confident of being able to give entire satisfaction in workmanship and price. I furnish or make the

Gold Mountings for Hair Jewelry

Of any style or pattern desired. I also furnish the braids separate from the mountings, or the two complete. Persons buying books and wishing to procure

BRAIDING TABLES, WEIGHTS, BOBBINS, MOLDS or FORMS,

Will be supplied at very low rates. For the accommodation of my trade, I have made arrangements to have Braiding Tools and materials

Manufactured in very large quantities,

Which I will furnish at prices sufficient only to cover the cost of manufacture and transportation.

M. CAMPBELL

MANUFACTURES

TOOLS AND MATERIALS

FOR ALL KINDS OF HAIR WORK.

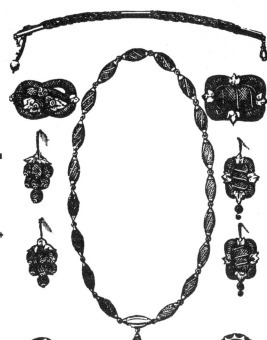

Hackles.

Weaving Cards.

Curling Irons.

Crimping Irons.

Forms.

Pinching Irons.

Curling Tongs

Gold Mountings.

ROOTING MACHINES,

FOR PLACING THE ROOTS OF COMBINGS ALL ONE WAY.

Price, from \$3 to \$15.

WEAVING STANDS.

Price, from \$2 to \$5.

BRAIDING TABLES.

Price, from \$2 to \$5.

BOBBINS AND WEIGHTS FOR BRAIDING.

APPENDIX

While the commercial production of hair work has virtually disappeared, there is renewed interest in "hairwork" as evidenced by the establishment of the *HAIR ART INTERNATIONAL RESTORERS (H.A.I.R.) SOCIETY* in 1992 and its growing membership. The society is dedicated to promoting and preserving the art of making beautiful things of human and animal hair and publishes a regular newsletter. For further information, the society can be contacted through Ruth Gordon, 24629 Cherry St., Dearborn, MI 48124.

As evidence of commercial hair work production today, the following is excerpted from a letter received by this publisher from Joanna Svensson of Sweden.

[Born in Chicago in 1935, Joanna later married a Swedish student and moved to Varnhus where she raised her family. With a background in art and music, her observations at Varnhus are most pertinent.]

"A couple of years after my arrival here at Vamhus, some of the ladies doing hairwork gave a class in the art. They were all growing old and many of them didn't really remember all the patterns...The old ladies held a few more classes which I joined... Since then, I have taught at least 16 classes in hair work. A rough guess is that about 20 ladies of our town do hairwork commercially today, most of it on order for those who wish to have a keepsake of their own or a relative's hair, but even for sale to tourists.

Here at Vamhus there was a local historical society... They collected things but had no place to show them and the old crafts were dying out. We rounded up some friends...and formed a tourist organization. Its purpose was among others to arrange daily demonstrations of our local crafts, hairwork and making chipwood baskets (of hand split slats). These demonstrations took place every day from Midsommmardagen, around June 25 to the middle of Aug. when the school term starts... The Hairworkers, who were willing to give of their time for almost no pay, sold their items or took orders... Now the Historical society finally has opened their museum and (for) the past 10 or 12 years, they have taken over these activities. People come from all over...the world, to see us do hairwork. Last summer I met a gentleman from Munich who was out buying old hairwork (and some new) for a museum to be opened there... There is a museum at Fredrikshavn in Denmark that also has a large exhibit of hairwork. Our local musesum has a large collection as well...

...I was amused to read that the art of hairwork has been zealously guarded as a profound secret. Yes, this is true. We only allow Vamhus people to partake in our classes. I was lucky to have learned it, but after all, we resided here. Among others, I have taught my own three daughters. The old ladies told us that we must never teach anyone not from here. That is because of the history.

We don't know who started to do hairwork here. In fact from the start, some decades before 1850, trading and working with hair was guarded by the Wigmakers guild and not allowed. Perhaps that is why our young women, once they had learned the craft, usually travelled to foreign countries, where they went from door to door or advertised their trade. They could be as young as 15 years the first season. The years when crops failed and there was a famine, whole families could leave for a period of hair working. Each year from this town of 2000 persons from 100 to 300 people could go off doing hair work. Since many of the workers were young and pretty, some married in other countries, Finland, Scotland, Germany Denmark and others. One or two of the ladies made such a success in London and Edinburough that they even delivered work to Queen Victoria and other royal persons. Hearsay has it that they also did work for the Czar of Russia. Many Swedish people lived and worked in St. Petersburg, so it wasn't strange for the hairworkers to go there either.

Now you know that hairwork has a living and unbroken tradition here at Vamhus and that we still do work commercially. I think we do it to an extent that is unprecedented anywhere else in the world. It has never been a sole livelihood for any except a very few (like the lady in London, but even she returned to farming at the next town, built a fine house and barn with the earnings.) Even today, hairwork is a second occupation, or a hobby for "pinmoney". Sometimes it is a meager earning for girls at college or for young unemployed mothers who can earn a little in spare mements."

Joanna Svensson, May 1993
Varnhus, Sweden